SpringerBriefs in Psychology

Advances in Child and Family Policy and Practice

Editor in Chief

Barbara H. Fiese, University of Illinois at Urbana-Champaign, Urbana, IL, USA

More information about this series at http://www.springer.com/series/10143

Julie Poehlmann-Tynan
Editor

Children's Contact with Incarcerated Parents

Implications for Policy and Intervention

Commentary by Karen P. Bogenschneider

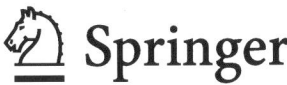

Editor
Julie Poehlmann-Tynan
Human Development & Family Studies
University of Wisconsin-Madison
Madison, WI, USA

ISSN 2192-8363 ISSN 2192-8371 (electronic)
SpringerBriefs in Psychology
ISBN 978-3-319-16624-7 ISBN 978-3-319-16625-4 (eBook)
DOI 10.1007/978-3-319-16625-4

Library of Congress Control Number: 2015938390

Springer Cham Heidelberg New York Dordrecht London
© Springer International Publishing Switzerland 2015
This work is subject to copyright. All rights are reserved by the Publisher, whether the whole or part of the material is concerned, specifically the rights of translation, reprinting, reuse of illustrations, recitation, broadcasting, reproduction on microfilms or in any other physical way, and transmission or information storage and retrieval, electronic adaptation, computer software, or by similar or dissimilar methodology now known or hereafter developed.
The use of general descriptive names, registered names, trademarks, service marks, etc. in this publication does not imply, even in the absence of a specific statement, that such names are exempt from the relevant protective laws and regulations and therefore free for general use.
The publisher, the authors and the editors are safe to assume that the advice and information in this book are believed to be true and accurate at the date of publication. Neither the publisher nor the authors or the editors give a warranty, express or implied, with respect to the material contained herein or for any errors or omissions that may have been made.

Springer International Publishing AG Switzerland is part of Springer Science+Business Media (www.springer.com)

Foreword

Advances in Child and Family Policy and Practice serves as a SpringerBriefs forum for discussion of issues related to social policy and services for children, adolescents, and their families with a particular emphasis on a psychosocial perspective. Each brief undergoes a rigorous peer review process and editorial review by the editor in chief. Further, each brief is grounded in the most up-to-date scientific evidence that enables researchers and stakeholders to translate research to practice and policy.

In this brief, Poehlmann-Tyan and colleagues highlight innovative and groundbreaking research documenting the family processes that occur following parental incarceration. Based in attachment and ecological theories, the authors pin-point how disruptions in parenting may be associated with children's adaptation to parental incarceration. Experiences during visitation under varying conditions (e.g., through Plexiglas or video visitations) are clearly detailed as are physiological responses to living arrangements prior to incarceration. The brief concludes with a commentary by a noted expert in family policy and recommendations for future research and policy implementation.

This brief is not only a practical resource for administrators and law enforcement and corrections personnel who have daily contact with parents who are incarcerated, but it also serves as a guide for future research. *Children's Contact with Incarcerated Parents* is an important read for educators and mental health professionals who work with the millions of children affected by incarceration. The brief details the clear and actionable steps that can be taken as the result of this research, thereby improving the well-being of numerous children.

Barbara H. Fiese
Editor in Chief, Advances in Child and Family Policy and Practice

Preface

Contact between incarcerated parents and their children has received increased attention because of its potential effects on child and adult relationships and well-being, parenting, and corrections-related issues, such as institutional behavior and recidivism. This brief presents an executive summary (Poehlmann-Tynan, 2015) and literature review on what we know about contact (Shlafer, Loper, & Schillmoeler, 2015) in addition to three new empirical papers, followed by a summary and commentary. The empirical papers focus on contact in both jail and prison settings. As jails in the United States handle almost 20 times more admissions per year than prisons, and studies of jailed parents and their children are not common in the literature, two of the studies focus on jails.

In the first chapter, Dallaire and colleagues examine whether 7- to 12-year-old children's contact with their jailed mothers is associated with children's self- and other-reported internalizing and externalizing behavior problems (Dallaire, Zeman, & Thrash, 2015). Findings suggest that more frequent contact through letters and phone calls was associated with fewer child internalizing problems, whereas more frequent visits, conducted through Plexiglas barriers at the jail, were associated with more internalizing problems.

In the second chapter, Poehlmann-Tynan and colleagues use observational methods to examine what happens during 2- to 6-year-old children's visits with jailed parents through Plexiglas barriers and video monitors (Poehlmann-Tynan et al., 2015). Findings suggest that children visually and verbally engaged with their incarcerated parents during visits, and they alternated between expressing positive emotions and being serious. Most children stayed in close proximity to their caregivers during their time at the jail, and they engaged in increasingly high levels of contact maintenance during the visit. Some aspects of the visit were unexpected, such as the amount of time children spent watching visits that occurred adjacent to them.

In the third chapter, McClure and colleagues present data from a multimethod exploratory investigation of 47 imprisoned mothers and their 4- to 12-year-old children, examining associations between mother and child contact, maternal cortisol levels, perceived parenting stress, and maternal adjustment (i.e., emotion dysregulation, depressive, and other mental health symptoms) at three timepoints (T1 at baseline, T2 before release, T3 6 months after release) (McClure et al., 2015). At T1, lower cortisol levels were found in mothers who lived with their children before incarceration compared to mothers who did not. At T3, more frequent mother–child contact was related to less recidivism.

Following the empirical chapters, a commentary explores what researchers needed to do to make effective policy recommendations.

Madison, WI, USA   Julie Poehlmann-Tynan, Ph.D.

Executive Summary

Children of Incarcerated Parents: A Growing and Vulnerable Population

Millions of US children experience the incarceration of a parent in prison or jail each year, and they are more likely to develop antisocial behavior and other problems compared to their peers. Although family relationships are important for incarcerated individuals, little attention has been paid to inmates' children. The children are not systematically identified, screened, or offered services, and typically they are not provided with supportive contexts for visiting their parents. High-quality research is scarce, and few caregiver resources exist to support children in their care. Children of incarcerated parents could benefit from systematic data collection documenting their numbers and needs over time; rigorous, focused, practical research to help inform policymakers and practitioners; caregiver support; and positive relationships with parents facilitated through family-friendly policies and practices during visits in prisons and jails.

Problem Description

The United States incarcerates more people than any other country in the world, and most incarcerated individuals are parents. Millions of children are affected, and they experience elevated risk for developing behavior problems in childhood, as well as physical and mental health difficulties as they grow up. Having contact with incarcerated parents, through visits, phone calls, and letters has long been deemed important for family well-being during and following incarceration, but few researchers, practitioners, and policymakers consider this issue from the child's viewpoint. We know that family visits are associated with decreased recidivism and improved institutional behavior for incarcerated individuals. Yet, what about the children?

Corrections facilities generally operate from a "safety and security" position, with little attention paid to visitors and their needs. The presence of families, and children in particular, is not usually considered. Compared to jails, prisons are more likely to offer face-to-face visits, although they increasingly rely on video visits. Compared to prisons, jails are more likely to offer visits behind Plexiglas or through video. More corrections facilities offer lower priced phone calls now than in the past, and sending letters through the mail remains a viable option for contact. However, few corrections facilities offer child-friendly visits, defined as providing safe and friendly environments for visits; fostering open communication among caregivers, children, incarcerated parents, and professionals about contact; adequately preparing children and adults for visits; facilitating parent–child contact between visits; and supporting incarcerated parents during the process (Dallaire, Poehlmann, & Loper, 2011).

New research presented by Dallaire, Zeman, and Thrash (2015) finds that, for children aged 7–12 years, more contact with jailed mothers via letters and phone calls is associated with fewer child symptoms such as withdrawal, sadness, and anxiety. Children can be reassured that their mother is safe and still loves them. However, more frequent visits, conducted through Plexiglas barriers at the jail, are linked with more anxiety symptoms in children. What happens during such visits that might be associated with anxiety? Observations of children aged 2–6 years during Plexiglas and video visits with jailed parents, conducted by Poehlmann-Tynan et al. (2015), reveal that children visually and verbally engage with parents. Most children stay in close proximity to their caregivers, increasingly as visits progress, suggesting needs for support. Many children spend time watching visits adjacent to them because of the lack of privacy. And consistent with previous research, McClure et al. (2015) find that more contact between imprisoned mothers and their children is linked with lower rates of recidivism for mothers.

Critique

Law enforcement and corrections are not only concerned with safety and security, prevention of crime, and punishment of offenders, but also with rehabilitation. Offering family visitation is one way to improve institutional behavior and decrease recidivism. We argue that it is also within the realm of public interest to support the children of incarcerated parents and their caregivers. Most corrections systems do not collect data on inmates' parental status, and other systems (e.g., child welfare, schools) typically do not have access to such data. As a result, our society is unaware of how many children are affected by parental incarceration or their elevated risk status. Moreover, rigorous research on children with incarcerated parents is still limited.

When visits to jails or prisons occur behind barriers or through video monitors, and children experience a lack of privacy when communicating with their parents, this may be stressful. Such feelings can interfere with the potentially positive effects of parent–child contact. Making the policies and process for contact more family-friendly and offering child-friendly visits may reduce children's anxiety while strengthening family relationships and still conferring benefits to inmates. Alternatives to visits, through phone calls and letters, are also important options to foster positive parent–child relationships within the context of corrections. Parent interventions also may facilitate positive contact and support reunification upon the parents' reentry.

Recommendation

The most compelling recommendation from the new studies and the existent body of research (see Poehlmann et al., 2010) is the need for understanding and supporting families within the context of corrections. Conducting rigorous research on affected families and offering child-friendly visits in corrections settings are key ways to do this. Implementing evidence-based parenting interventions and improving institutional policies and procedures that make them more family-friendly, including training corrections personnel to interact positively with families, are important. Supporting the adults who care for children with incarcerated parents is critical and may reduce the children's risk experiences.

A first, low-cost step to facilitate these types of improvements is to have corrections facilities systematically collect data on inmates' parental status through their intake or assessment process. Several states, including Oregon, have already required state corrections to do this. Making public system data easily available to researchers, and collaboration across states in this effort, is also critical. For example, Washington State has a web-based portal that makes such de-identified data available to the public (www.partnersforourchildren.org). Such data collection has shown that national figures underestimate the number of children affected by parental incarceration and calls attention to the needs of some of the most vulnerable members of our society. Integration and collaboration across systems are important as well because many children with incarcerated parents are involved with other systems (e.g., child welfare). The federal government has recognized that this issue does not neatly fit into one agency's portfolio and thus has established an interagency working (sub)group for children of incarcerated parents. Although this is an important step, support for family research in the context of corrections is also urgently needed.

Contents

1. **Introduction and Literature Review: Is Parent–Child Contact During Parental Incarceration Beneficial?** 1
   Rebecca J. Shlafer, Ann Booker Loper, and Leah Schillmoeller

2. **Differential Effects of Type of Children's Contact with Their Jailed Mothers and Children's Behavior Problems** 23
   Danielle Dallaire, Janice Zeman, and Todd Thrash

3. **Young Children's Behavioral and Emotional Reactions to Plexiglas and Video Visits with Jailed Parents** 39
   Julie Poehlmann-Tynan, Hilary Runion, Cynthia Burnson, Sarah Maleck, Lindsay Weymouth, Kierra Pettit, and Mary Huser

4. **Associations Among Mother–Child Contact, Parenting Stress, and Mother and Child Adjustment Related to Incarceration** 59
   Heather H. McClure, Joann Wu Shortt, J. Mark Eddy, Alice Holmes, Stan van Uum, Evan Russell, Gideon Koren, Lisa Sheeber, Betsy Davis, J. Josh Snodgrass, and Charles R. Martinez Jr.

5. **Children's Contact with Incarcerated Parents: Summary and Recommendations** 83
   Julie Poehlmann-Tynan

6. **Policy Commentary: The Research Evidence Policymakers Need to Build Better Public Policy for Children of Incarcerated Parents** 93
   Karen Bogenschneider

Index 115

About the Editor

Julie Poehlmann-Tynan, Ph.D. is a Professor in the Human Development and Family Studies department at the University of Wisconsin-Madison; director of the Center for Child and Family Well-Being at the University of Wisconsin; an investigator at the Waisman Center, an affiliate of the Institute for Research on Poverty; and a licensed psychologist. Through numerous publications and outreach efforts, she has brought the attention of the child development and family studies communities to the issue of parental incarceration. Her research with children of incarcerated parents has been funded by the National Institutes of Health and the Department of Health and Human Services. Dr. Poehlmann-Tynan has served as an advisor to Sesame Street to help develop and evaluate their Emmy-nominated initiative for young children with incarcerated parents and their families called Little Children, Big Challenges: Incarceration.

Contributors

Karen Bogenschneider University of Wisconsin-Madison, Madison, WI, USA

Cynthia Burnson Human Development & Family Studies, University of Wisconsin-Madison, Madison, WI, USA

Danielle Dallaire Integrated Science Center, The College of William & Mary, Williamsburg, VA, USA

Betsy Davis Oregon Research Institute, Eugene, OR, USA

J. Mark Eddy School of Social Work, University of Washington, Seattle, WA, USA

Alice Holmes Oregon Social Learning Center, Eugene, OR, USA

Mary Huser Cooperative Extension Family Living Programs, University of Wisconsin-Extension, Madison, WI, USA

Gideon Koren The Ivey Chair in Molecular Toxicology, Western University, London, ON, Canada

Ann Booker Loper University of Virginia, Charlottesville, VA, USA

Sarah Maleck Human Development & Family Studies, University of Wisconsin-Madison, Madison, WI, USA

Charles R. Martinez Jr. Center for Equity Promotion, University of Oregon, Eugene, OR, USA

Department of Educational Methodology, Policy and Leadership, University of Oregon, Eugene, OR, USA

Heather H. McClure Center for Equity Promotion, University of Oregon, Eugene, OR, USA

Kierra Pettit Human Development & Family Studies, University of Wisconsin-Madison, Madison, WI, USA

Julie Poehlmann-Tynan Human Development & Family Studies, University of Wisconsin-Madison, Madison, WI, USA

Hilary Runion Human Development & Family Studies, University of Wisconsin-Madison, Madison, WI, USA

Evan Russell Department of Medicine, Western University, London, ON, Canada

Leah Schillmoeller University of Minnesota, Minneapolis, MN, USA

Lisa Sheeber Oregon Research Institute, Eugene, OR, USA

Rebecca J. Shlafer Department of Pediatrics, University of Minnesota, Minneapolis, MN, USA

Joann Wu Shortt Oregon Social Learning Center, Eugene, OR, USA

J. Josh Snodgrass Department of Anthropology, University of Oregon, Eugene, OR, USA

Todd Thrash Integrated Science Center, The College of William & Mary, Williamsburg, VA, USA

Stan Van Umm Department of Medicine, Western University, London, ON, Canada

Lindsay Weymouth Human Development & Family Studies, University of Wisconsin-Madison, Madison, WI, USA

Janice Zeman Integrated Science Center, The College of William & Mary, Williamsburg, VA, USA

Chapter 1
Introduction and Literature Review: Is Parent–Child Contact During Parental Incarceration Beneficial?

Rebecca J. Shlafer, Ann Booker Loper, and Leah Schillmoeller

In 2007, more than 1.75 million children under the age of 18 had a parent in a state or federal prison in the United States (U.S.) (Maruschak, Glaze, & Mumola, 2010). Nationally, about 53 % of men and 61 % of women in U.S. prisons are parents (Maruschak et al., 2010). In 2007, this represented nearly 810,000 incarcerated parents, with a disproportionate number from racial minority backgrounds. Jails in the U.S. handled more than 11 million admissions in 2013, similar to the previous year (Minton & Golinelli, 2014), and many jailed inmates are parents as well. A recent report revealed that 1 in 28 children in the U.S. have an incarcerated parent, up from 1 in 125 children just 25 years ago (The Pew Charitable Trusts, 2010).

A growing body of research confirms that children with incarcerated parents are more likely than other children to exhibit internalizing (e.g., depression, anxiety, withdrawal) and externalizing (e.g., delinquency, substance use) behavior problems, cognitive delays, difficulties in school, and insecure attachment relationships with their incarcerated parents and primary caregivers (Eddy & Poehlmann, 2010). Here, and throughout this monograph, "caregiver" is used to refer to whoever serves as the child's primary caregiver during the parent's incarceration. When the incarcerated parent is the child's father, the primary caregiver is often the child's mother (Glaze & Maruschak, 2008). In contrast, when mothers are incarcerated, children often reside with a grandparent or another relative

R.J. Shlafer, Ph.D. (✉)
Department of Pediatrics, University of Minnesota, 717 Delaware Street SE,
Rm. 382, Minneapolis, MN 55414, USA
e-mail: shlaf002@umn.edu

A.B. Loper, Ph.D.
University of Virginia, Charlottesville, VA, USA

L. Schillmoeller, B.S.
University of Minnesota, Minneapolis, MN, USA

(Glaze & Maruschak, 2008). Thus, throughout this monograph the term "caregiver" is used to refer to whoever provides a majority of the daily care for the child during the parent's incarceration, recognizing that in some cases this is the child's biological parent.

Analyses using the Adverse Childhood Experiences database have shown increased long-term risk for multiple health problems in individuals who, as children, experienced the incarceration of a household member (e.g., Anda, Brown, Felitti, Dube, & Giles, 2008; Ford et al., 2011; Gjelsvik, Dumont, & Nunn, 2013). While we do not have a definitive understanding of the specific developmental pathways that lead to these adverse outcomes, it is plausible that positive contact and healthy communication patterns and relationships between inmate parents and their children could mitigate such problems.

1.1 Variations in Correctional Institutions

Often "parental incarceration" is used as an umbrella term, referring to incarceration in jail or prison. There are important differences, however, in these types of correctional facilities. Jails are locally operated correctional facilities (i.e., administered by cities or counties) that generally confine persons before or after the judicial decision or sentence, or house inmates for relatively short sentences. Sentences to jail are typically for misdemeanor offenses and usually last 1 year or less. Sentences to prison are typically for felony offenses and are generally more than 1 year (U.S. Department of Justice, http://www.bjs.gov/index.cfm?ty=tda, 2010), although a few states have combined jail and prison systems. While there may be similarities between individuals incarcerated in both jails and prisons (e.g., mental health problems, history of substance use, poverty), there are also important differences. In comparison to county jails, prisons generally house more serious offenders, for longer periods of time, and prisons often have the space, infrastructure, and staff to provide a wider array of services for inmate rehabilitation (e.g., remedial education, chemical health treatment, parenting education).

There are also differences between state prisons, where an individual is incarcerated for breaking a state law, such as driving under the influence or selling drugs on the street, and federal prisons where an individual is incarcerated for breaking a federal law, such as money laundering, insider trading, or running a drug cartel. In comparison to jails, prisons—particularly federal prisons—are often located farther from the inmate's residence at the time of arrest. The type of facility (i.e., county jail, state prison, federal prison) has important implications for children and families. The type of facility can impact the inmates' proximity to their families, the probable frequency of contact, as well as the format and rules for contact and visitation. Although some federal and state laws guide the broad rules for contact and visitation, administrators within corrections departments in individual states and counties also write policies; even within one jurisdiction, visiting policies may vary by facility.

1.2 Variations in Contact by Facility Type

1.2.1 Contact with Jail Inmates

In order to better understand the likely sources of variability both between and within the varying types of institutions, we collected public information regarding types of contact from selected institutions. For our analysis, we selected jails by identifying the most populous county in each state, and then identified one jail that served each county (e.g., Fulton County Jail, Georgia). A total of 50 jails were identified and contact procedures were examined. The type of visitation was recorded from available information on public websites and then ascertained through phone calls by undergraduate research assistants to each jail. Research assistants called the primary phone number listed on the jail's public website and inquired about the types of visits children could have with an incarcerated parent (i.e., "What type of visiting can children have with their parents at this facility?"). Results are summarized in Table 1.1 and Fig. 1.1.

For 11 jails (22 %), information about the type of visitation was available on the jail's website. We were able to gather additional information by phone from 90 % of jails. We were unable to obtain information on visiting types from three jails, despite repeated attempts to call the primary phone number listed on each jail's website. Among the 50 jails surveyed, six jails permitted two types of visits (e.g., barrier and video visits). Across all 50 jails, barrier visits were the most common ($n=30$, 60 %), 10 (20 %) jails utilized on-site video visits, 8 (16 %) jails utilized off-site video visits, and 7 (14 %) offered face-to-face or contact visits. One jail (Milwaukee County) did not allow children under the age of 18 to visit. Clearly in jail settings, face-to-face visits are uncommon across the U.S.

1.2.2 Contact with State Prisoners

A recently published report includes detailed state-by-state information related to visitation policies and identifies commonalities and variation in visitation policies, including accessibility of visiting policies online, availability of written policies, and information on specific procedures and rules for visiting (Boudin, Stutz, & Littman, 2012). To date, this is the most comprehensive and accurate review of visitation policies within state corrections systems across the country.

We built on this work by reviewing visitation types for individual state prisons. Because policies and visitation types can vary by facility even within the same state's department of corrections (Boudin et al., 2012), we restricted our search to the prison with the largest inmate population (based on available data, such as daily inmate reports) in each state. Our process for ascertaining information about visiting types in state prisons was similar to our approach with jails. We started by recording information publically available on the facilities' or states' department of

Table 1.1 Visitation type for one county jail(s) in the most populous county in each state (November 2013)

State	Most populous county	Jail name	Visitation type
Alabama	Jefferson	Jefferson County Jail	Barrier
Alaska	Anchorage	Anchorage Correctional Complex	Barrier / Video (on-site)
Arizona	Maricopa	Durango Jail	Contact[a]
Arkansas	Pulaski	Pulaski County Regional Detention Facility	Barrier
California	Los Angeles	Men's Central Jail	Barrier / Video
Colorado	El Paso	Criminal Justice Center	Video (off-site)[a]
Connecticut	Fairfield County	Bridgeport Correctional Center	Barrier
Delaware	New Castle County	Howard R. Young Correctional Institution	Barrier[a] / Contact
Florida	Miami-Dade County	Turner and Guilford Knight Correctional Center	Barrier[a]
Georgia	Fulton County	Fulton County Jail	Video (off-site)[a]
Hawaii	City and County of Honolulu	Oahu Community Correctional Center	Contact[a] / Barrier
Idaho	Ada County	Ada County Jail	Video (off-site)[a]
Illinois	Cook County	Cook County Jail	Barrier[a]
Indiana	Marion County	Marion County Jail	Barrier
Iowa	Polk County	Polk County Jail	Video (off-site)
Kansas	Johnson County	Johnson County Jail	Barrier / Video (on-site)
Kentucky	Jefferson County	Louisville Department of Corrections	Video (on-site)
Louisiana	East Baton Rouge Parish	East Baton Rouge Parish County Jail	Barrier
Maine	Cumberland County	Cumberland County Jail	Barrier
Maryland	Montgomery	Montgomery County Detention Center	Barrier
Massachusetts	Middlesex	Middleton House of Corrections	Barrier
Michigan	Wayne	Division 1: The Andrew C. Baird Detention Facility	Barrier
Minnesota	Hennepin	Hennepin County Jail (Adult Detention Center)	Barrier[a]
Mississippi	Hinds	Hinds County Farm Penal Jail	Contact
Missouri	St. Louis	St. Louis County Jail (The Buzz Westfall Justice Center)	Barrier
Montana	Yellowstone County	Yellowstone County Detention Center	Barrier

(continued)

1 Introduction and Literature Review: Is Parent–Child Contact During Parental...

Table 1.1 (continued)

State	Most populous county	Jail name	Visitation type
Nebraska	Douglas County	Douglas County Jail/Douglas County Correctional Center	Video (on-site)
Nevada	Clark County	Clark County Detention Center	Video (on-site)[a]
New Hampshire	Hillsborough County	Hillsborough County Jail	Barrier
New Jersey	Bergen County	Bergen County Jail	Barrier
New Mexico	Bernalillo County	Metropolitan Detention Center	Video (on- & off-site)[a]
New York	Kings County	Kings County Jail	Video (on-site)
North Carolina	Mecklenburg County	Mecklenburg County Jail-Central	No information
North Dakota	Cass County	Cass County Jail	Barrier
Ohio	Cuyahoga County	Cuyahoga County Corrections Center	Barrier
Oklahoma	Oklahoma County	Oklahoma County Jail	Video (on- & off-site)
Oregon	Multnomah County	Inverness Jail	Barrier
Pennsylvania	Philadelphia County	Philadelphia Detention center	Contact
Rhode Island	Providence County	Anthony P. Travisono Intake Service Center	Contact
South Carolina	Greenville County	Greenville County Detention Center	No information
South Dakota	Minnehaha County	Minnehaha County Jail	Video (on- & off-site)
Tennessee	Shelby County	Shelby County Jail	Barrier Contact
Texas	Harris County	Harris County Jail	Barrier
Utah	Salt Lake County	Salt Lake County Jail/Metro Jail	Barrier
Vermont	Chittenden	Chittenden Regional Correctional Facility	No information
Virginia	Fairfax	Fairfax County Virginia Adult Detention Center	Barrier
Washington	King	King County Adult Detention Center	Barrier
West Virginia	Kanawha	South Central WV Regional Jail & Correctional Facility Authority	Barrier
Wisconsin	Milwaukee	Milwaukee County Jail	None
Wyoming	Laramie	Laramie County Detention Center	Video (on-site)

[a]Information available about visitation types available online

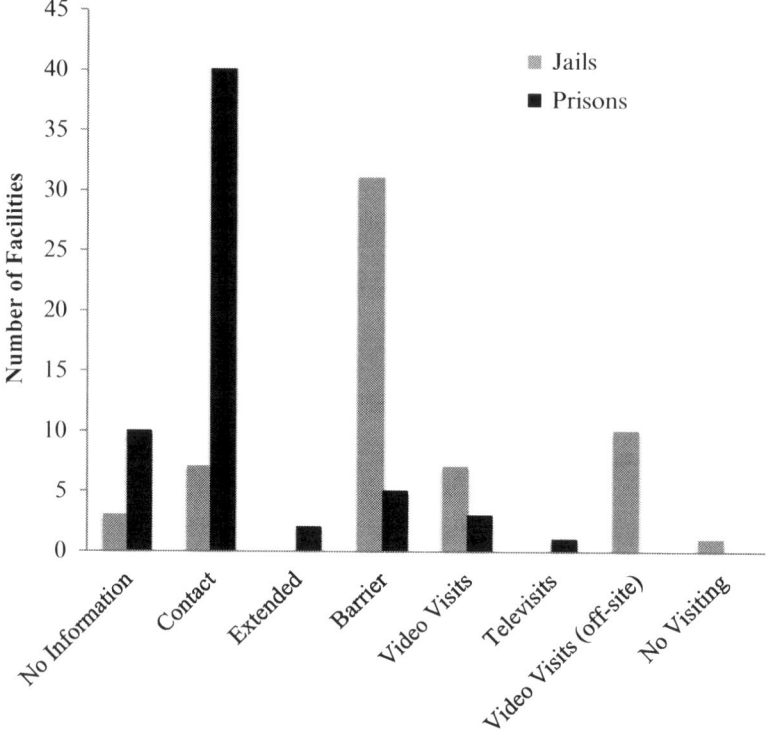

Fig. 1.1 Types of visits in selected state prisons (N = 50) and county jails (N = 50) (November 2013)

corrections websites. If information was not available on the websites, an undergraduate research assistant contacted the facilities by phone using the number that was listed on the facilities' public webpage. Results are summarized in Table 1.2 and Fig. 1.1.

We were unable to obtain information through the website or by phone about the type of visitation permitted at ten prisons. Among the remaining 40 prisons that we searched and contacted by phone, all facilities permitted contact visits between incarcerated parents and their children. Ten (25 %) of the 40 facilities with available information listed more than one visitation type (e.g., contact visits and extended visits).

1.2.3 Contact with Federal Prisoners

The United States Bureau of Prisons (BOP) regulates contact and visitation with inmates in federal prisons. By law, a federal prisoner is allowed at least 4 h of visiting time per month, though often individual facilities can provide additional time.

1 Introduction and Literature Review: Is Parent–Child Contact During Parental... 7

Table 1.2 Visitation type for largest state prison in each state (November 2013)

State	Number of state prisons	Prison name	Visitation type
Alabama	15	Limestone Correctional Facility	Contact
Alaska	13	Goosecreek Correctional Institution	Contact
Arizona	10	Arizona State Prison Complex—Lewis	Contact; extended visits
Arkansas	18	Cummins Unit	Contact
California	34	Wasco State Prison	Contact; extended visits
Colorado	19	Sterling Correctional Facility	No information
Connecticut	18	MacDougall-Walker Correctional Institution	No information
Delaware	4	Sussex Correctional Institution	No information
Florida	64	Blackwater River Correctional Facility	No information
Georgia	23	Calhoun State Prison	No information
Hawaii	4	Halawa Correctional Facility	Contact
Idaho	8	Idaho Correctional Center	Contact
Illinois	27	Stateville Correctional Center	Contact
Indiana	19	Miami Correctional Facility	Contact
Iowa	7	Newton Correctional Facility	Contact
Kansas	7	Ellsworth Correctional Facility	Contact
Kentucky	8	Luther Luckett Correctional Complex	Contact
Louisiana	10	Louisiana State Penitentiary	Contact
Maine	6	Maine State Prison	Contact
Maryland	15	Central Maryland Correctional Facility	Contact
Massachusetts	14	Massachusetts Correction Institution: Norfolk	Contact
Michigan	36	Michigan Reformatory	Contact
Minnesota	9	Minnesota Correctional Facility—Faribault	Contact[a]
Mississippi	3	Mississippi State Penitentiary	No information
Missouri	19	Jefferson City Correctional Center	Contact
Montana	5	Montana State Prison	Contact
Nebraska	8	Tecumseh State Correctional Institution	Contact[a]
Nevada	7	High Desert State Prison	No information
New Hampshire	3	New Hampshire State Prison for Men	Contact
New Jersey	11	South Woods State Prison	Contact
New Mexico	6	Penitentiary of New Mexico	Contact[a]
New York	52	Clinton Correctional Facility	Contact
North Carolina	66	Scotland Correctional Institution	Contact; barrier
North Dakota	3	North Dakota State Penitentiary	Contact; video visits
Ohio	22	Chillicothe Correctional Institution	Contact; video visits

(continued)

Table 1.2 (continued)

State	Number of state prisons	Prison name	Visitation type
Oklahoma	17	Lexington Assessment & Reception Center/Lexington Correctional Center	Contact
Oregon	14	Snake River Correctional Institution	Contact
Pennsylvania	26	SCI Graterford	Contact
Rhode Island	7	John J. Moran Medium Security Facility	Contact
South Carolina	26	Kershaw Correctional Institution	No information
South Dakota	6	Mike Durfee State Prison	Contact; barrier
Tennessee	11	West Tennessee State Penitentiary	Contact; barrier
Texas	50	Coffield	No information
Utah	2	Utah State Prison (Draper)	Contact; Barrier
Vermont	7	Northern State Correctional Facility (NSCF)-Newport	Contact
Virginia	34	Greensville Correctional Center	Contact; barrier and video visits
Washington	12	Coyote Ridge Corrections Center	Contact
West Virginia	11	Huttonsville Correctional Center	No information
Wisconsin	20	Oshkosh Correctional Institution	Contact; televisits
Wyoming	3	Wyoming Medium Correctional Institution	Contact

[a]Non-contact visits for inmates with restrictions (e.g., crimes against children)

Prison administrators may also limit the length of visits or the number of people who can visit at one time, in order to avoid overcrowding in the visiting room. Visiting regulations are available through the BOP website (www.bop.gov/policy/progstat/5267_008.pdf); the program statement includes the technical and legal language set forth by the BOP regarding visiting. In addition, the BOP has recently added a user-friendly guide to visiting on their website (http://www.bop.gov/inmates/visiting.jsp).

1.2.4 Variations in the Types of Contact

Positive contact and healthy communication between incarcerated parents and their children can help maintain or even enhance the quality of the parent–child relationship. However, there is considerable variation in the frequency and type of contact that incarcerated parents can have with their children, and such variation may have important implications for the impact of contact on children's outcomes. Below we summarize three primary types of contact: letter-writing, phone calls, and visits.

1.2.5 Letter-Writing

Letter-writing is the most frequent vehicle for parent–child contact, with an estimated 52 % of parents in state prisons having at least monthly mail contact with at least one of their children (Glaze & Maruschak, 2008). There are several reasons for this apparent preference: letters are inexpensive, they can be saved and re-read, and they involve few logistics pertinent to correctional settings (e.g., personal searches). For the inmate, there is time to reflect on the content of the letter before sending, and for the receiving child, there is the opportunity to hear from the parent in the familiar home setting. The child can opt whether or not to read the letter and, when needed, caregivers can monitor the messages being delivered. However, a potential downside of letter writing is the lack of immediacy. In a letter, the child may not have the opportunity to talk about the day's events and then receive the parent's reactions within the likely timeframe that the event is of importance. A parent's letter about a great test grade or winning ball game may be old news to the child by the time it is read. Further, very young children are dependent on their caregivers for both letter-reading and letter-writing, although they may be able to draw pictures for the incarcerated parent.

1.2.6 Email

Recent initiatives allow email contact between inmates and their loved ones; however, the rules and restrictions vary by facility and not all facilities have systems in place for this type of contact. All BOP operated facilities utilize the Trust Fund Limited Inmate Computer System (TRULINCS) application, which enables the exchange of secure electronic messages between inmates and individuals in the community (http://www.bop.gov/inmates/trulincs.jsp). All individuals in the community must be on the inmates' approved contact list and persons in the community may approve or choose to block the inmates' messages. The TRULINCS system allows for inmates to send and receive electronic messages. Email has some of the same advantages as regular mail (e.g., allowing time to reflect on the content, allowing caregivers to monitor contact), and may also allow for more timely communication. However, the type of media that can be sent is often limited (e.g., restrictions on attachments like pictures, inability to print content to keep). Some facilities allow offenders to send, but not receive, messages. Other facilities print email correspondence and delivered to inmates by institutional staff. These restrictions obviously limit many of the advantages of email.

Another potential advantage is cost, as electronic messages are often less expensive than the postage and supplied (e.g., paper, envelope) required to send a letter in the mail. The costs vary by vendor and facility, and are based upon agreements with the correctional agencies. For instance, the CorrLinks system charges inmates in Iowa $0.25 per message and inmates in Minnesota $0.30 per message (https://www.

corrlinks.com/FAQ.aspx#Answer12). JPay, another vendor that offers a number of services to inmates and their families (e.g., sending money to the inmate, phone calls, video visits) has a different fee structure. Individuals in the Branchville Correctional Facility in Indiana, for example, are charged $4.00 for 10 email postage "stamps", where each typed page of text costs one "stamp" and attachments cost an additional "stamp" (https://www.jpay.com/Facility-Details/Indiana-Department-of-Correction/Branchville-Correctional-Facility.aspx). Thus, even though the costs may be less expensive than regular postage, costs are still incurred by inmates and may prevent some families from being able to connect in this way.

1.2.7 Phone Calls

The second most frequent medium for communication between incarcerated parents and their children is via the telephone. An estimated 38 % of parents in state prisons have at least monthly phone contact with their children (Glaze & Maruschak, 2008). As with letter-writing, phone calls have inherent advantages and disadvantages. Phone calls can allow parents to communicate in real time and get immediate feedback on how a child is responding. As with a letter, a child receives a phone call within the security and familiarity of home.

However, phone calls also present a host of challenges. Depending upon the institution, phone calls can be very expensive (Greene 2013). Recently the U.S. Federal Communication Commission (FCC) adopted a plan to set maximum rates for calls in jails and prisons that are below the very high rates usually encountered by families of prisoners in the past (FCC, 2012, 2013). However, specific rules for this policy are still underway, and possible legal challenges may affect implementation (Sledge, 2013).

Another challenge is with the physical set-up for phone calls in most institutions, which involves a bank of phones on a wall, sometimes with small side partitions. This set-up often makes it difficult for inmates to hear or be head, and to discuss sensitive matters with their loved ones. Calls are typically time-limited, forcing family members to triage how the costly time is spent among those who wish to talk. Moreover, young children depend on support from their caregivers to participate in meaningful phone calls.

1.2.8 Personal Visits

Although much of the public may view personal visits as the typical form of parent–child contact for prisoners and jai inmates, visits personal visits are rare for most inmates, with an estimated 60 % of both mothers and fathers in state prisons reporting that they never receive visits (Glaze & Maruschak, 2008). The personal visits that do occur can take multiple forms. Until recent years, visitation has been

1 Introduction and Literature Review: Is Parent–Child Contact During Parental...

limited to either face-to-face visits in which inmates and family members meet in a common space (sometimes referred to as "contact visits", despite limited physical contact often allowed), or barrier visits in which inmates are separated by a glass wall (i.e., Plexiglas). A recent innovation for personal visitation is the use of extended visits, in which visitation is integrated with parenting training and inmates have longer visitation sessions, during which physical contact and child engagement is encouraged. In addition to these forms of personal visitation, new technological innovations have afforded a variety of video or virtual forms of contact. As with letter-writing and phone calls, each of these contexts affords special benefits and limitations.

1.2.9 Face-to-Face Visits

Face-to-face visits are arguably the most desired by inmates who often view separation from family as the most difficult of prison stressors (e.g., Celinska & Siegel, 2010; Foster, 2012; Mignon & Ransford, 2012). The physical set-up for such visits can vary considerably across institutions. While there is no unitary prototype for face-to-face visits, they frequently take place in a large room that accommodates multiple families. In many corrections facilities, such visits take place across a low table, with chairs on either side. Under optimal visitation arrangements, children can see and interact with their parents and be assured first-hand of their parents' safety, and multiple family members can be together in a supportive milieu.

This type of visit is also commonly referred to as a "contact visit"; however, depending upon the security requirements, inmates may be prohibited from touching or holding their children. Facilities may vary in terms of the availability of child-centric toys or activities. Prior to having a face-to-face visit, children may undergo personal searches, and facilities may have regulations that limit when and with whom visits are allowed. Nesmith and Ruhland (2008) interviewed 34 children regarding their experiences associated with having a parent in prison and observed several fearful views regarding prison visitation. For example, one child reported, "It's got a lot of doors you can't open. There's this desk with two guards. They call us over…You can't get up, but if you say you had to go to the bathroom, you can't go back in there (p.1126)." The hospitality and child-centric atmosphere of a face-to-face visit may moderate child outcomes associated with such contact (Poehlmann, Dallaire, Loper, & Shear, 2010).

1.2.10 Enhanced Visits

Some facilities offer opportunities for inmates and their children to have face-to-face or contact visits in a family-friendly environment. Some facilities offer this type of enhanced visiting experience to inmates concurrently participating in a parenting program, as is the case for women participating in Extended Visiting at the Minnesota Correctional Facility—Shakopee. As outlined by the Minnesota Department of Corrections, the purpose of Extended Visiting is to provide offenders with "additional visiting privileges in order to build and/or maintain a nurturing relationship with their own children during the extended visits." Incarcerated mothers currently assigned to the Anthony Unit, a privileged living unit within the facility, are eligible to participate in Extended Visiting if they have children under the age of 17 years old. Compared to standard visits, these extended visits are longer (approximately 3 h) and take place in a child-friendly environment. During these visits, mothers and their children participate in structured and unstructured activities, including arts and crafts, free play in the gymnasium, and lunch. Rules for extended visits are notably different than standard, face-to-face visits in the visiting room. For example, a number of items are allowed in the facility for extended visit that would otherwise be prohibited, including additional children's clothing, diapers and wipes, formula, and baby bottles or sippy cups. Rules for physical contact between inmates and their children are also different between standard and extended visits. During standard visits, for example, only a brief hug and kiss on the cheek at the beginning and end of the visit are allowable. In contrast, during extended visits, mothers are allowed to have additional physical contact with their own children, including kisses, hugging, and hand-holding.

According to Boudin et al. (2012), at least six other states have policies that allow for enhanced or extended visiting (e.g., overnight family visits, 4- or 8-h visits in a child-oriented or family-like setting). These types of visitation are uncommon and little is known about the different types of enhanced visits that facilities offer or how such visits are incorporated into existing parenting programming. Future research should examine incarcerated parents', caregivers', and children's perceptions of enhanced visits and how this unique type of face-to-face visit impacts children's outcomes.

1.2.11 Barrier Visits

In contrast to personal visits in which inmates can touch and interact with inmates, some facilities utilize a Plexiglas wall to separate visitors. Barrier visits are typically implemented when there is heightened safety concern, such as in jails or high-security prisons. Thus, the primary advantage to children in these venues is the heightened protection, as they are not exposed to the inmate population and the visitor screening may be somewhat less intrusive than that for face-to-face meetings. The disadvantages are usually associated with uncomfortable contexts that are less child-friendly. Since facilities usually have limited stations for these visits, visitors may wait long periods in a holding area for their turn to visit a loved one. Depending upon the time of year (e.g., the winter holidays), there can be heavy traffic for visits that translates into longer waiting periods. The physical set-up in these cases typically involves a series of stations separated by partitions, often with a single stool that is bolted to the floor. Conversation is heard either via holes in the partition or by a phone hook-up. The physical arrangement can restrict meaningful contact between children and parents, as children cannot touch or be held by parents. Limited furnishing may mean that a child either sits on the caregiver's lap, stands aside, shares the available chair, or sits on a shelf in front of the Plexiglas window. In a survey that included 211 visitors to a county urban jail that provided barrier visitation, Sturges and Al-Khattar (2009) found that approximately two-thirds were dissatisfied with the visitation room. Specific complaints revolved around the inability to have physical contact, the lack of privacy, and uncomfortable chairs.

1.2.12 Virtual Visits

Virtual or video visitation is a recent addition to the facilities for contact between inmates and their family members. In a video visit, an inmate interacts with family or friends through a computer or telecommunications network that enables real-time visual and audio connection. The supporting technology and usage varies between highly restricted and secure systems that require specialized equipment, to systems that use existing Internet applications. In many cases private vendors, such as JPay, set up web-based or closed circuit camera kiosks in correctional facilities that enable inmates to speak, often for a fee, with friends and family (http://www.jpay.com/PVideoVisit.aspx). Depending upon the fee structure, the correctional facility can gain additional revenue from video visits (Eickhoff, 2010). The fees for video visits can vary widely (Phillips, 2012). Whereas some facilities offer video visits at no cost to the inmates or their visitors, others charge a flat fee per visit or per minute. The Dakota County Jail in Minnesota, for instance, does not charge for video visits if the visitors come to the jail, but visitors who wish to connect from home are charged $.50/min (or $10 for the 20 min visit). In contrast, through a contract with JPay, the Indiana Department of Corrections charges $9.95 for 30 min of video visitation (http://www.jpay.com/PVideoVisit.aspx).

The most restrictive type of virtual visitation is via closed-circuit telecommunication equipment. With this arrangement, family members come to the facility and view the inmate through a television or computer monitor that is connected to equipment used by the inmate. This set-up essentially duplicates the glass barrier, but substitutes an electronic communication arrangement. As with the barrier visit, the arrangement has generally good security and reduced visitor screening. Correctional facilities may prefer this version of contact as it conserves the need for correctional staff, limits movement within the institution, and conserves space (Emmanuel, 2012). However, for family members, these visits may represent the intersection of disadvantages of other forms of contact. These visits require the travel and expense of coming to the institution, may involve uncomfortable waiting periods, and afford limited opportunities for child-friendly interaction. In a survey that included 70 visitors to a suburban jail that employed video visitation, approximately two-thirds indicated dissatisfaction with the practice (Sturges & Al-Khattar, 2009).

In contrast to the closed-circuit video visitation described above that is becoming increasingly evident in many jails, a number of prisons have become interested in video visitation that enables contact with family members who do not travel to the institution. For this type of contact, inmates' family members either go to a regional center that has the needed computer equipment (e.g., a local library or a community center), or alternately they use personal devices from their own home.

With community-based video visitation, children can see and hear parents in real time and potentially engage in meaningful activities. For example, the Osborne Association is a New York City community-based provider that offers video visits, or televisits, in a child-friendly setting to children with a parent at Albion or Clinton Correctional Facilities in upstate New York (personal communication, A. Hollihan, Osborne Association televisiting program manager, November 12, 2013). Participating mothers complete Osborne's parenting program and are offered a support group to discuss their televisiting successes and challenges. Fathers participate in a televisiting parenting workshop and individual coaching sessions with parents are facilitated by Osborne's community-based instructor via videoconference. Children and caregivers are also provided with support.

With community-based video visitation, children do not have to travel great distances or endure security procedures. These visits can offer unique benefits not available in other contact settings (Loper & Coleman, 2014). For example, parents and children can do homework together and work on common art projects. The inmate parent can receive immediate coaching on how to engage their children. At the same time, caregivers and visiting children can be supported by the staff at the collaborating community agencies that are committed to helping families affected by incarceration. Difficulties of this set-up tend to revolve around logistic problems of gaining transportation to the community centers and coordinating with prison staff to schedule visits. The equipment used for the visit may also affect the quality of contact. A small kiosk with an attached handset, a typical installation with private vendors, likely does not afford the more natural milieu created by the use of equipment with an internal 'hands-free' microphone, a larger screen, and nearby toys, puppets, and books with which to engage children.

An alternative to this arrangement is one in which families use their own home computers or electronic devices to contact their incarcerated family member. This arrangement can be attractive to families as it further reduces travel and logistic difficulties and can enable easier scheduling of visits. Much like a phone call, the inmate can theoretically 'visit' with greater flexibility. The downside of this approach is the potential loss of the opportunity for family to make connections with a supportive community agency. In addition, the costs of either community- or home-based video visitation may be prohibitive for some families. While the recent FCC ruling (2012, 2013) seeks to rein in costs associated with inmate phone calls, to our knowledge there has not been any similar consideration of limits on video visitation fees. Moreover, some corrections facilities have not moved to use of home computers for virtual visits because of concerns about security and confidentiality.

1.3 Contact Between Children and Incarcerated Parents: Is it Beneficial?

For inmates in jails or prisons, contact with loved ones plays a pivotal role in their lives. Many inmates eagerly await the phone calls, letters, and visits that keep them connected to the outside. There is good evidence that keeping such connections can help. For example, frequent visitation with family members has been linked to better post-release outcomes (Bales & Mears, 2008), frequent phone and letter contact has been linked to less perceived parenting stress during incarceration (Loper, Carlson, Levitt, & Scheffel, 2009), and higher levels of contact during prison relate to an inmate's self-reported attachment to children after release (La Vigne, Naser, Brooks, & Castro, 2005). The body of work that attests to the importance of home and family connections for returning inmates (Travis, Solomon, & Waul, 2001; Visher & Courtney, 2007) affords a convincing rationale for why family contact can be beneficial to inmates. However, there is much less research regarding the benefits of such contact for children.

When parents are incarcerated, there is typically a significant shift in the amount of child contact. In a review of multiple surveys undertaken by the Bureau of Justice Statistics (BJS), Maruschak et al. (2010) emphasize the change and upheaval in children's home arrangements that occur following parental arrest and incarceration. Based on a BJS survey, prior to imprisonment, a majority of mothers and nearly half of fathers resided with at least one child, with approximately three-quarters of mothers and one fourth of fathers serving as the primary childcare provider (Glaze & Maruschak, 2008). Most parents in state prisons reported maintaining some form of contact with their children during the parent's imprisonment. However, the frequency and type of contact changes markedly over time, with fewer than half of parents reporting any type of weekly contact with children during the first year after admission. Further, contact is most typically via phone or letters, and only 8 % of the inmates report weekly personal visits with children (Maruschak et al., 2010).

In the relatively little available research that links contact with incarcerated parents and child outcomes, findings tend to point to potential benefits of inmate parent–child contact. For example, Loper et al. (2009) reported that more frequent letter-writing to children by fathers and mothers in prison was associated with a better co-parenting alliance with the child's caregiver, a context that other studies have associated with better child outcomes (Gasper, Stolberg, Macie, & Williams, 2008).

In a study of 94 incarcerated mothers of young children, Poehlmann (2005a) reported that more frequent phone contact with children was linked to mothers' perceptions of a better relationship between themselves and their children. Trice and Brewster (2004) observed that adolescents with incarcerated mothers who had frequent contact with their mothers were less likely to drop out of school.

However, other studies give pause to any sweeping generalization regarding benefits of contact. For example, in a study that included children of jail inmates,

Dallaire, Ciccone, and Wilson (2012) found that more frequent phone calls, letters, and visits were associated with problematic "role-reversal" themes in children's family drawings. This pattern, in which children expressed a sense of responsibility for caring for their incarcerated parent was not evident in the drawings of a control sample of children separated from their parents for other reasons. Shlafer and Poehlmann (2010) interviewed 57 caregivers and children who largely reported problematic depictions of personal visitation experiences. Caregivers expressed concerns about exposing children to the prison environment and voiced a need to protect children from potentially negative interactions with imprisoned parents. In a similar vein, Poehlmann (2005b) detected a trend in which children who had not recently visited their mothers in prison had more secure attachment representations of their mothers and caregivers.

In a review of the literature focusing on contact between children and their incarcerated parents, Poehlmann et al. (2010) argued that the effects of parent–child contact could not be globally described as good or bad. Rather, they argued that such effects depend on variations in the quality of visitation experiences. From this lens, each type of contact that is available to inmate parents and their families involves varying contextual features that are relevant to how such contact is experienced by children and other family members. As described earlier in this chapter, the characteristics of the correctional facility and the specific type of contact are two contextual features that have important implications for how children experience contact with their incarcerated parents. Understanding institutional variability and the differences between specific types of contact can inform common problems and potential solutions needed to promote positive child outcomes in the context of parental incarceration.

1.4 Challenges of Making Contact: Implications for Families

Most institutions have policies for enabling contact between incarcerated parents and their children. The impetus for this stems, in part, from the well-documented body of work that attests to the importance of family connection for positive inmate adjustment before and after prison (Visher & Courtney, 2007). However, families who wish to take advantage of contact experiences may not always be able to reap the intended benefits. The varying types of contact that are available each have specific benefits and limitations that impact contact quality and families' experiences. Moreover, as we found in our search for information about individual policies, institutions can vary widely in the types of contact permitted, and sometimes this information can be difficult to locate.

In addition to these considerations, our examination of various institutions provided insight into the difficulties inmates' families may face when they seek to learn about contact opportunities. While many of the websites had *some* information about visiting, the sites were often difficult to navigate. In some instances, information about visiting was available, but it was difficult to find or not presented in a user-friendly way. Very few websites, for instance, provided information about the types of visits (i.e., face-to-face, barrier, video) or the security procedures that children and families could expect to experience at the facility, thereby making it difficult to prepare family members for the visitation process.

Gathering information from county or state websites was also challenging because the sites frequently changed. During the course of this project, for instance, the Minnesota Department of Corrections rolled out a new website. The new site offered more information and was easier to navigate; it contained additional information about contact with inmates, including specific considerations for children and families. It is impossible to know if other states are in the process of improving their sites or changing the policies as we have documented them here.

As an inmate's family member might do, we also sought to clarify information via phone. However, despite multiple attempts to call phone numbers that were listed online, there were some jails and prisons that could not be reached. In some instances, when we reached staff via telephone, we were met with considerable resistance. Some staff members were unwilling to answer basic questions about the type of visiting available or specific rules for children. Sometimes staff indicated that visitation information was only available for people who were already on an inmate's visitation list. Other staff were unprofessional. For example, when we asked about the type of visits children could have with their parents at one county jail, a staff member said "Are you knocked up? Because if you are knocked up, you can just visit. But, if you've had the baby, then you need a birth certificate."

Whereas the challenges we encountered gathering the information may limit our understanding of the type of visits offered by a range of corrections facilities across the U.S. from a research perspective, it is also a serious concern for families trying to work within the system. The lack of available information makes it difficult for caregivers, as well as professionals, working with families to help prepare and support children for visits.

1.5 Overview of the Monograph

Contact is an important aspect in the lives of prisoners and their families, but the benefits of this contact can vary widely depending upon critical contextual features. Three questions that can inform our understanding of this complex issue are:

1. Knowing that the type of contact inmates can have with their families can take many forms—phone, mail, visits—are there discernable differences in children's outcomes by contact-type? In Chap. 2, Dallaire, Zeman, and Thrash (2014) examine whether children's (7–12 years) contact with their jailed mothers was associated with children's self- and other-reported internalizing and externalizing behavior problems. Findings suggest that more frequent contact via letters

and phone calls was associated with fewer internalizing problems, whereas more frequent in-person contact via barrier visitation was associated with more internalizing problems.
2. Today, most of the inmates in the U.S. are in jails. Given that most jails ascribe to non-contact visitation procedures (e.g., barrier and video visits), how do young children react when visiting their parents in these contexts? In Chap. 3, Poehlmann-Tynan et al. (2014) look more in-depth at the process of children's visits with incarcerated parents when barrier and video visits are used. They present observational data regarding young children's (2 to 6 years) emotional and behavioral reactions to visiting their parents in jail settings. Findings suggest that children engaged with their incarcerated parents during the visit and alternated between expressing positive emotions and being serious. Most children stayed in close proximity to their caregivers during the visit and engaged in an increasingly high level of contact maintenance during the visit. Some aspects of the visit were unexpected, such as the amount of time children spent watching visits that occurred adjacent to them.
3. How does contact between children and their incarcerated mothers relate to maternal and child adjustment during and after incarceration? In Chap. 4, McClure, Shortt, Eddy, Holmes, Van Uum, Russell et al. (2014) present data from a multimethod exploratory investigation of 47 incarcerated mothers and their children (age 4–12 years) examining associations between mother-child contact, maternal cortisol levels, parenting stress, and child and maternal adjustment (i.e., child behavior problems, and maternal emotion dysregulation, depressive and other mental health symptoms) at three timepoints (T1 at baseline, T2 before release, T3 6 months after release). The benefits of mother-child contact on maternal stress at T1 were indicated by the lower cortisol levels for mothers who lived with their children before incarceration compared to mothers who did not. At T3, increased mother-child contact was related to reduced recidivism as indicated by a decreased likelihood of detention within 6 months after release. More contact was related to higher levels of internalizing symptoms in children, although types of contact could not be disaggregated because of the nature of the data collected.

Following the empirical chapters, a summary and recommendations for intervention and policy are presented by Poehlmann-Tynan (2014). A policy commentary by Bogenschneider (2014) explores what researchers need to do to make effective policy recommendations in this area of family scholarship, suggesting that more high-quality research is needed. The monograph concludes with a policy brief focusing on the family-related needs of children with incarcerated parents.

Acknowledgements Dr. Shlafer's time on this publication was supported by the National Center for Advancing Translational Sciences of the National Institutes of Health Award Number UL1TR000114. The content is solely the responsibility of the authors and does not necessarily represent the official views of the National Institutes of Health.

References

Anda, R. F., Brown, D. W., Felitti, V. J., Dube, S. R., & Giles, W. H. (2008). Adverse childhood experiences and prescription drug use in a cohort study of adult HMO patients. *BMC Public Health, 8*, 198.

Bales, W. D., & Mears, D. P. (2008). Inmate social ties and the transition to society: Does visitation reduce recidivism? *Journal of Research in Crime & Delinquency, 45*, 87–321. doi:10.1177/0022427808317574.

Bogenschneider, K. P. (2014). The research evidence policymakers need to build better public policy for children of incarcerated parents. In J. Poehlmann-Tynan (Ed.), *Children's contact with incarcerated parents: Implications for policy and intervention. Advances in child and family policy and practice*. New York: Springer.

Boudin, C., Stutz, T., & Littman, A. (2012). Prison visitation policies: A fifty state survey. *Yale Law School, Public Law Working Paper*.

Celinska, K., & Siegel, J. (2010). Mothers in trouble: Coping with actual or pending separation from children due to incarceration. *The Prison Journal*. Published on-line at http://tpj.sagepub.com/content/90/4/447 doi:10.1177/0032885510382218

Dallaire, D., Ciccone, A., & Wilson, L. C. (2012). The family drawings of at-risk children: Concurrent relations with contact with incarcerated parents, caregiver behavior and stress. *Attachment & Human Development, 14*(2), 161–183. doi:10.1080/14616734.2012.661232.

Dallaire, D. H., Zeman, J., & Thrash, T. (2014). Differential effects of type of children's contact with their jailed mothers and children's behavior problems. In J. Poehlmann-Tynan (Ed.), *Children's contact with incarcerated parents: Implications for policy and intervention. Advances in child and family policy and practice*. New York: Springer.

Eddy, J. M., & Poehlmann, J. (Eds.). (2010). *Children of incarcerated parents: A handbook for researchers and practitioners*. Washington, DC: Urban Institute Press.

Eickhoff, T. J. (2010, May 25). Video visitation: Evolving revenue streams. *Correctional News*. Retrieved from http://www.correctionalnews.com/articles/2010/05/25/video-visitation-evolving-revenue-streams

Emmanuel, A. (2012, August 7). In-person visits fade as jails set up video units for inmates and families. New York Times. Retrieved from http://www.nytimes.com/2012/08/07/us/some-criticize-jails-as-they-move-to-video-visits.html?smid=pl-share

Federal Communications Commission. (2012, December 28). In the matter of rates for interstate inmate calling services: Notice of proposed rulemaking. Retrieved from http://hraunfoss.fcc.gov/edocs_public/attachmatch/FCC-12-167A1.pdf

Federal Communications Commission. (2013, August 9). FCC reduces high long-distance calling rates paid by inmates. Retrieved from https://www.fcc.gov/document/fcc-reduces-high-long-distance-calling-rates-paid-inmates

Ford, E. S., Anda, R. F., Edwards, V. J., Perry, G. S., Zhao, G., Li, C., et al. (2011). Adverse childhood experiences and smoking status in five states. *Preventive Medicine, 53*(3), 188–193.

Foster, H. (2012). The strains of maternal imprisonment: Importation and deprivation stressors for women and children. *Journal of Criminal Justice, 40*, 221–229. doi:10.1016/jcrimjus.2012.01.005.

Gasper, J. A. F., Stolberg, A. L., Macie, K. M., & Williams, L. J. (2008). Co-parenting in intact and divorced families: Its impact on young adult adjustment. *Journal of Divorce & Remarriage, 49*, 272–290. doi:10.1080/10502550802231924.

Gjelsvik, A., Dumont, D. M., & Nunn, A. (2013). Incarceration of a household member and Hispanic health disparities: Childhood exposure and adult chronic disease risk Behaviors. *Preventing Chronic Disease, 10*, 120281. doi:http://dx.doi.org/10.5888/pcd10.120281

Glaze, L., & Maruschak, L. (2008). Parents in prison and their minor children. Bureau of Justice Statistics Special Report. Washington, DC: U.S. Department of Justice. Retrieved from http://www.bjs.gov/content/pub/pdf/pptmc.pdf

Greene, J. (July 2013). FCC tackles cost of prison phone calls. *The Blog of Legal Times.* Retrieved from http://legaltimes.typepad.com/blt/2013/07/fcc-tackles-cost-of-prison-phone-calls.html

La Vigne, N. G., Naser, R. L., Brooks, L. E., & Castro, J. L. (2005). Examining the effect of incarceration and in-prison family contact on prisoners' family relationships. *Journal of Contemporary Criminal Justice, 21*(4), 314–335. doi:10.1177/1043986205281727.

Loper, A. B., Carlson, L. W., Levitt, L., & Scheffel, K. (2009). Parenting stress, alliance, child contact, and adjustment of imprisoned mothers and fathers. *Journal of Offender Rehabilitation, 48*(6), 483–503. doi:10.1080/10509670903081300.

Loper, A. B. & Coleman, E. (2014, March/April). Video visitation for inmates: Thinking outside of the tiny box. *Corrections Today*, 54–59.

Maruschak, L. M., Glaze, L., & Mumola, C. (2010). Incarcerated parents and their children: Findings from the Bureau of Justice Statistics. In J. M. Eddy & J. Poehlmann (Eds.), *Children of incarcerated parents* (pp. 189–216). Washington, DC: The Urban Institute.

McClure, H. H., Shortt, J. W., Eddy, J. M., Holmes, A., Van Uum, S., Russell, E., et al. (2014). Associations among mother-child contact, parenting stress, hair cortisol, and mother and child adjustment related to incarceration. In J. Poehlmann-Tynan (Ed.), *Children's contact with incarcerated parents: Implications for policy and intervention. Advances in child and family policy and practice.* New York: Springer.

Mignon, S., & Ransford, P. (2012). Mothers in prison: Maintaining connections with children. *Social Work in Public Health, 27,* 69–88. doi:10.1080/19371918.2012.630965.

Minton, T. D., & Golinelli, D. (2014). *Jail inmates at midyear 2013: Statistical Tables.* Bureau of Justice Statistics. Washington, DC: U.S. Department of Justice.

Nesmith, A., & Ruhland, E. (2008). Children of incarcerated parents: Challenges and resiliency in their own words. *Children and Youth Services Review, 30*(10), 1119–1130. doi:10.1016/j.childyouth.2008.02.006.

The Pew Charitable Trusts. (2010). *Collateral costs: Incarceration's effect on economic mobility.* Washington, DC: The Pew Charitable Trusts.

Phillips, S. (2012). Video visits for children whose parents are incarcerated: In whose best interest? Report for The Sentencing Project. Retrieved from http://sentencingproject.org/doc/publications/cc_Video_Visitation_White_Paper.pdf

Poehlmann, J. (2005a). Incarcerated mothers' contact with children, perceived family relationships, and depressive symptoms. *Journal of Family Psychology, 19,* 350–357. doi:10.1037/0893-3200.19.3.350.

Poehlmann, J. (2005b). Representations of attachment relationships in children of incarcerated mothers. *Child Development, 76*(3), 679–696. doi:10.1111/j.1467-8624.2005.00871.x.

Poehlmann, J., Dallaire, D., Loper, A. B., & Shear, L. D. (2010). Children's contact with their parents in prison: Research findings and recommendations. *American Psychologist, 65,* 575–598. doi:10.1037/a0020279.

Poehlmann-Tynan, J. (2014). Children's contact with their incarcerated parents: Summary and recommendations. In J. Poehlmann-Tynan (Ed.), *Children's contact with incarcerated parents: Implications for policy and intervention. Advances in child and family policy and practice.* New York: Springer.

Poehlmann-Tynan, J., Runion, H., Burnson, C., Maleck, S., Weymouth, L., Pettit, K., et al. (2014). Young children's behavioral and emotional reactions to plexiglas and video visits with jailed parents. In J. Poehlmann-Tynan (Ed.), *Children's contact with incarcerated parents: Implications for policy and intervention. Advances in child and family policy and practice.* New York: Springer.

Shlafer, R. J., & Poehlmann, J. (2010). Attachment and caregiving relationships in families affected by parental incarceration. *Attachment & Human Development, 12,* 395–415. doi:10.1080/14616730903417052.

Sledge, M. (2013). Prison phone call industry will fight new FCC rules lowering rates for inmates. Huffington Post September 2, 2013. Retrieved from http://www.huffingtonpost.com/2013/09/09/prison-phone-call-fcc_n_3894556.html

Sturges, J., & Al-Khattar, A. (2009). Survey of jail visitors about visitation policies. *The Prison Journal, 89*, 482–496. doi:10.1177/0032885509351009.

Travis, J., Solomon, A., & Waul, M. (2001). *From prison to home: The dimensions and consequences of prisoner reentry*. Washington, DC: The Urban Institute Press.

Trice, A. D., & Brewster, J. (2004). The effects of maternal incarceration on adolescent children. *Journal of Policy and Criminal Psychology, 19*, 27–35. doi:10.1007/BF02802572.

U.S. Department of Justice, Bureau of Justice Statistics. Terms and definitions. Retrieved March 26, 2015, from http://www.bjs.gov/index.cfm?ty=tda.

Visher, C., & Courtney, S. (2007). *One year out: Experiences of prisoners returning to Cleveland*. Washington, DC: The Urban Institute Press.

Chapter 2
Differential Effects of Type of Children's Contact with Their Jailed Mothers and Children's Behavior Problems

Danielle Dallaire, Janice Zeman, and Todd Thrash

The question of what type of contact, if any, best serves the psychological and emotional needs of children who are separated from their mothers and fathers because of parental incarceration remains a topic in need of empirical inquiry. Although contact may offer distinct benefits to the incarcerated parent (e.g., recidivism, Bales & Mears, 2008), impacts on children's psychological well-being are not well understood (Poehlmann, Dallaire, Loper, & Shear, 2010). Shlafer and Loper (this issue) highlight that there is considerable complexity with regard to understanding the impact of contact with an incarcerated parent and that particular attention should be given to the different types of contact children have with their incarcerated parent, including letter-writing, phone calls and personal visits.

Maintaining contact with an incarcerated parent may help maintain relationship bonds and enable children to feel connected to their incarcerated parent who may be an important attachment figure. However, previous research indicates that non-contact barrier visits with incarcerated parents may undermine children feelings of safety and security (Dallaire, Ciccone, & Wilson, 2012; Pohelmann, 2005). In middle childhood, children may manifest their insecurity with symptoms of anxiety and depression (Brumariu & Kerns, 2010). Although some studies have suggested that contact visits between incarcerated parents and their children that occur as part of a parent-education program have beneficial effects (e.g., Purvis, 2013), most children with parents incarcerated in jail facilities do not have the opportunity to have a contact visit with their parent (Poehlmann et al., 2010, see also Shlafer & Loper, this issue). In the current study we focus more broadly on the impact of non-contact

D. Dallaire (✉) • J. Zeman • T. Thrash
Integrated Science Center, Room 1143, College of William and Mary, Williamsburg, VA 23187-8795, USA
e-mail: dhdall@wm.edu

barrier visits on children's internalizing and externalizing behavioral problems. Non-contact visits with an incarcerated mother may be associated with greater internalizing and externalizing behavior problems as children may experience feelings of sadness, anxiety or helplessness after seeing their mother and not being afforded the opportunity to be comforted by physical contact (Arditti, Lambert-Shute, & Joest, 2003). Children may also act out or externalize such feelings, as there may be comorbidity between internalizing and externalizing behavior problems (see Lilenfeld, 2003). We do not expect other forms of contact to be associated with greater internalizing or externalizing behavior problems, to the contrary, previous research would suggest that other forms of contact may help children (Dallaire, Ciccone, & Wilson, 2010) and parents (Tuerk & Loper, 2006) process the difficult emotions they may be feeling during the separation.

Further, although the assumption is that some contact is better than no contact with an incarcerated parent, empirical examination of this question is warranted. In an investigation of youth between 4 and 15 years of age, Shlafer and Poehlmann (2010) found that lack of contact with an incarcerated parent was associated with greater feelings of alienation toward that parent. We seek to replicate and extend that finding by examining if lack of contact with an incarcerated mother is associated with internalizing and externalizing behavior.

The few studies to investigate how contact with incarcerated parents affects child psychological adaptation have added important preliminary information to our knowledge base but are limited in a variety of ways that are representative of the broader literature on children with incarcerated parents (for a review see Shlafer & Loper, this issue and Poehlmann et al., 2010). First, most research on children of incarcerated parents has examined the effects of paternal incarceration on children, with few studies examining the specific outcomes associated with maternal incarceration (Murray, Farrington, & Sekol, 2012) which may confer unique, significant stressors for children (Dallaire, 2007). Second, the use of small sample sizes which preclude the capability to conduct sophisticated analyses (Murray et al., 2012) that can uncover or highlight the complex web of findings characterize this research area. Third, further compounding the small sample size issue is the reliance on a single reporter and single method design. Research has generally relied on mother or caregiver report of children's behaviors (Tuerk & Loper, 2006) although teacher perceptions have also been used (Dallaire et al., 2010). Fourth, in some studies (e.g., Dallaire, Ciccone, & Wilson, 2012), the developmental stage of the child has not been considered but rather a wide range of ages from preschool through adolescence has been analyzed as one developmental period. It is likely that the impact of parental incarceration may differ depending on the developmental competencies of the child. Fifth, samples have often combined jail and prison samples, although they differ in several important ways (Poehlmann & Eddy, 2013). Finally, when examining how contact with an incarcerated parent affects children, research has typically not distinguished among the various types of contact (personal visits, mail contact) with the parent. The examination of visits versus phone calls and letters with the incarcerated parent may yield different outcomes. Further, although at least one study has found that some contact is better than no contact with an incarcerated parent (Shlafer & Poehlmann, 2010), further empirical examination of this question is warranted.

In the current study, we were interested in understanding whether contact with incarcerated mothers was associated with children's psychological functioning as indexed by internalizing and externalizing symptoms. Research has indicated that children experiencing maternal incarceration may exhibit psychological problems due to the associated stressors of this life event (e.g., Dallaire, Zeman, & Thrash, 2015), as well as family instability (e.g., Maruschak, Glaze, & Mumola, 2010). We were particularly interested in whether psychological maladaptation would be buffered by different forms of contact with mothers in jail. We chose the developmental period of middle childhood (7–12 years) to study because it is during these years that many social, emotional, and cognitive skills are being refined and solidified to ideally form the foundation to weather some of the stresses associated with adolescence (Shiner, 1998). It is also during this stage that parents continue to exert important socializing influences on children's development prior to the onset of the increasing power of the peer group (Zeman, Cassano, & Adrian, 2013). Thus, contact with incarcerated mothers during this period may be particularly important to children as they face the transition to adolescence.

Not only did we examine general contact with mothers while in jail, but we delved into this topic by examining the unique effects of barrier visits in the jail setting versus phone calls and letters versus no contact. In doing so, we addressed some of the aforementioned limitations by using a large sample of children in the middle childhood age range (7–12 years) whose mothers were incarcerated in jail at the time of the study. We obtained reports from multiple informants including children, their caregivers, and their mothers in order to provide a variety of perspectives on children's experiences of contact with their incarcerated mothers and children's behavior problems. Finally, the use of structural equation modelling permitted a rigorous examination of the interplay among these variables.

Based on the limited literature base, we formulated and tested three hypotheses. First, we hypothesized that, in comparison to a differentiated construct of contact based on visits and other forms of contact, the construct of global contact (i.e., all types of contact included in one latent variable) would not produce as strong a model fit due to the wide variation in the specific effects associated with visits versus other forms of contact. Second, we expected that children's visits with their incarcerated mother would be associated with greater internalizing and externalizing behavioral difficulties than other forms of contact. We expected other types of contact to be associated with lower levels of internalizing and externalizing behavior. Third, we hypothesized that having no contact of any type with one's incarcerated mother would be associated with greater internalizing and externalizing behavioral patterns. However, we anticipated that the findings for the third hypothesis may be affected by the reasons for the lack of contact (i.e., lower SES, more family instability) and thus, may moderate the associations to the psychological outcomes.

2.1 Method

2.1.1 Participants

The initial sample consisted of 236 jailed mothers, with the final sample consisting of interviews completed with 118 caregivers[1] of 156 children. Because some children ($n=9$) were unaware of their mother's incarceration, only data from the 147 children who knew that their mothers were incarcerated are analyzed here. Thus, participants included 147 children of 114 jailed mothers[2] and 118 caregivers (for additional information about participant retention see Dallaire et al., 2015). Children (53.6 % boys) ranged in age from 78.20 months (6.50 years)—155.80 months (12.98 years) with a mean age of 9.80 years (118.05 months ($SD=20.01$ months)). Most children self-identified themselves as African American (61.7 %) and 29.8 % self-identified as Caucasian.

Children's mothers ranged in age from 24 to 50 years of age ($M=32.85$ years, $SD=5.91$ years), and on average, mothers had three biological children (range 1–7). If mothers had multiple children in the eligible age range, each child participated (see more below). In total, 41.7 % of children ($n=58$) had a sibling participate in the current study. The mother sample was ethnically diverse (64.1 % African American, 36.8 % Caucasian) and many reported low education, with 35.1 % reporting that they had not completed 12th grade or the high school equivalency exam. Mothers' report of their socioeconomic status (SES; Hollingshead, 1957) was in the low range ($M=1.68$, $SD=1.01$, range 1–4). Mothers were incarcerated for various reasons including contempt of court (including parole violations, 31.6 %), property crimes (e.g., larceny, 27.2 %), substance abuse issues (e.g., prescription fraud, distribution of illegal substances, 16.7 %), and other less frequently reported reasons like fraud (e.g., identity theft, 12.3 %) and violent crimes (e.g., armed robbery, 6.1 %). The number of times mother had been incarcerated ranged from 1 to 11 ($M=2.65$, $SD=1.64$) with 25.0 % of mothers reporting their first incarceration.

The 118 caregivers (74.8 % female) included children's grandparents (61.9 %), their fathers (18.0 %), other relatives (e.g., aunt, sibling, 17.3 %), and step-parents (2.9 %). They ranged in age from 19 to 70 years of age ($M=47.75$ years, $SD=11.56$ years) and although 28.3 % reported not completing 12th grade, 21.0 % had taken some college courses and 9.5 % had graduated from college. Caregivers' reports of their socioeconomic status (SES; Hollingshead, 1957) was in the low range ($M=2.03$, $SD=1.14$, range 1–5).

---

[1] The term "caregiver" is used broadly to refer to the person taking care of the child during the mother's incarceration.

[2] Analyses presented in this paper were also performed on a smaller sample of 114 mother-child and caregiver triads which only included one child chosen at random from the family and does not include siblings. The results are essentially the same and are available upon request.

2.1.2 Procedure

After receiving IRB approval from the authors' university's protection of human subjects committee, cooperating jail facilities reviewed and approved the research protocol. Recruitment and data collection occurred over a 2-year period. Women incarcerated at one of six Virginia jail facilities were recruited to participate by project staff. Project members went directly into housing cells and/or pods and described the project and asked eligible women to sign up to participate. Eligibility recruitments included having at least one child within the specified age range (7–12 years), having maintained parental rights, and no documented history of abuse or neglect to the target child. If a mother had multiple children in the age range, they were interviewed on separate occasions about each participating child. Mothers participated by completing a privately conducted one-on-one interview with the research assistant at the jail facility. Mothers provided consent for researchers to contact the child's caregiver along with information about how to contact the child's caregiver. Due to IRB concerns about the potential for coercion, mothers were not compensated for their participation.

After contact was made with a caregiver, interviews were scheduled at the caregiver's convenience. Interview locations included participants' homes (80.0 %), local libraries (16.0 %), other public locations (e.g., McDonalds, 2.0 %), and university lab facilities (2.0 %). After caregiver consent and child assent was obtained, participants went to separate locations to complete the hour-long interview. Caregivers and children were remunerated for their time.

2.1.3 Measures

Socioeconomic Status (SES). The Hollingshead Four Factor Index of Social Status (Hollingshead, 1957) was calculated based on Maternal and Caregiver education levels and occupations. The Hollingshead social strata system has been shown to have good validity (Deonandan, Campbell, Ostbye, Tummon, & Robertson, 2001). Raw scores can range from 8 to 66 and are grouped into five strata representing increasing levels of SES (with lower values indicating lower SES). In the present study, each child's SES stratum was based on the average of the mother's and caregiver's SES stratum score ($M=1.81$, $SD=0.83$; range: 1–4).

Contact with the Incarcerated Mother. Mothers and caregivers provided information about frequency of contact, including letter writing, phone calls and visitation with the target child. Mothers rated their frequency of phone, mail, and in person contact with the child using a 10-point scale with $1 = never/no\ contact$ to $10 = daily/weekly\ contact$ (10 = weekly in the case of visitation), the scale midpoint of $5 = Once\ every\ 3\ months$. In addition, children also reported if they had visited their mother at jail in the previous month (*Yes/No*). Interactions between mothers and their children were categorized as involving visits or phone calls and letters.

In the jail setting, no direct physical contact was permitted and visits occurred behind Plexiglas barriers.

We also created variables to capture a lack of contact between mothers and children based on caregiver's report. We choose to utilize caregiver report because mother's might be motivated to tell us that they were in current contact with their child so as not to be excluded from participating, further, given the lapse between mother and caregiver interviews, the caregiver report was more recent. A total of 26 caregivers (17.7 %) reported that children did not have any contact with their incarcerated mothers.

Children's Internalizing and Externalizing Behavior: Mother and caregiver report. Mothers and caregivers reported on children's internalizing and externalizing behavior problems over the previous 6 months using the Child Behavior Checklist (CBCL; Achenbach & Rescorla, 2001). The CBCL contains 113 items and yields three broad-band scales and eight syndrome scales. Only the internalizing and externalizing scales were used in the current study. Validation studies indicate strong internal consistency with adequate content, criterion-related, and construct validity (Achenbach & Rescorla, 2001). In the current study, internal consistencies for Internalizing and Externalizing problems were strong for mothers/caregivers (Internalizing: $\alpha=.86/.86$, Externalizing: $\alpha=.74/.81$). According to mothers'/caregivers' reports, respectively, 20.8 %/17.2 % of children were in the clinical range for Internalizing problems whereas 29.2 %/25.2 % of children were in the clinical range for Externalizing problems.

Internalizing Symptoms: Child report. Children's report of depressive symptomatology was assessed using the Children's Depression Inventory (CDI; Kovacs, 1992). Due to IRB concerns, the suicide item was omitted. The psychometric properties of the CDI have been well established and are acceptable (Carey, Gresham, Ruggiero, Faulstich, & Enyart, 1987). Within this sample, raw scores ranged from 0–36 ($M=8.08$, $SD=7.03$) with 6 children (3.97 %) meeting the clinical cut-off (T-score >65) and 35 children (18.2 %) receiving total raw scores of 13 or higher, indicating mild to moderate levels of depression (Kazdin, 1989; Smucker, Craighead, Craighead, & Green, 1986). Internal consistency was strong ($\alpha=.84$).

Children's anxious symptomology was assessed with the Multidimensional Anxiety Scale for Children (MASC; March, 1997). This measure yields a global score as well as four subscales including physical symptoms (tense/restless and somatic/autonomic), social anxiety (humiliation/rejection and public performance fears), harm avoidance (perfectionism and anxious coping), and separation/panic. Children responded to the 39 items using a 4-point Likert scale. The MASC has demonstrated excellent internal reliability, test-retest reliability, and validity (Baldwin & Dadds, 2007; March, 1997). In the current study the total score was used and items demonstrated strong internal consistency ($\alpha=.88$).

Externalizing Behaviors: Child report. Children's report of externalizing behavior was assessed with the 38-item Risky Behavior Protocol (RBP, Conger, Elder, Lorenz, Simons, & Whitbeck, 1994) that contains two subscales: 19-items that evaluate behaviors the child has done ("things you do"), and 19 items assess behaviors the child's friends have done ("things your friends do"). Only the "things you do" subscale was used in the current study. The items assess both major risk-taking and delinquency (e.g., purposely set fire in a building or in any other space), minor risk-taking (e.g., ridden in a car without a seat belt), and any risk-taking behavior (e.g., smoked cigarettes or used tobacco). Children indicate on a 3-point scale the frequency of the behavior. This instrument has acceptable internal consistency and validity (Rudasill, Reio, Stipanovic, & Taylor, 2010). In our sample, internal consistency was strong ($\alpha = .88$) and scores ranged from 0 to 29 ($M = 4.31$, $SD = 4.08$).

To determine whether children victimize (bully) others, children completed four items from the Engagement in Bullying Behavior subscale of the Kids in my Class at School questionnaire (Ladd, Kochenderfer, & Coleman, 1996, 1997). Using a 5-point Likert scale, children respond to four questions such as "Do you pick on other kids in your class at school?" "Do you hit other kids in your class at school?" Research has demonstrated acceptable internal validity (Ladd et al., 1996; Perdue, Manzeske, & Estell, 2009). For the current study, the measure showed acceptable internal reliability (Cronbach's $\alpha = .78$).

2.2 Results

2.2.1 Descriptive and Preliminary Data Analyses

Descriptive data for all study variables are presented in Table 2.1. Because child age and gender were associated with other study variables (e.g., CBCL-Int, CBCL-Ext, MASC) they were entered as control variables in all subsequent analyses. Additional control variables included child ethnicity (Black/non-Black) and SES. Black children were less likely to have mail contact with their mother (according to mother report) and to have lower levels of internalizing behavior (caregiver-report only) and externalizing behavior (mother and caregiver reports). SES was correlated with children's bullying behavior.

Mothers' and caregivers' reports of contact between the child and the incarcerated mother are presented in Table 2.2. Although mothers' and caregivers' reports were significantly, positively correlated (rs range from .39–.74, ps < .01), paired samples t-tests indicated significant differences between mothers' and caregivers' reports of phone contact and visitation. Specifically, mothers reported more phone contact than did caregivers, whereas caregivers reported more visits than did mothers.

2.3 Primary Analyses

Given that we obtained child, mother, and caregiver report of most variables, we used structural equation modeling (SEM) to disentangle structural effects among latent constructs from correlations resulting from reporter-specific method variance. Analyses were conducted using Amos version 20 (Amos Development Corp.,

Table 2.1 Descriptive data and correlations

	1	2	3	4	5	6	7	8	9	10	11	12	13	14	15	16	17	18	M (SD)
1. Age	–																		118.05 (20.00)
2. Gender[a]	–.09	–																	0.46 (0.50)
3. Ethnicity[b]	.06	–.02	–																0.59 (0.49)
4. SES[c]	–.04	.07	.13	–															4.18 (0.85)
5. Letter-M[d]	–.06	.15	–.21*	.17	–														5.57 (3.79)
6. Letter-C[e]	–.11	.11	–.11	.14	.39**	–													5.88 (3.68)
7. Phone-M	.06	.11	–.07	.12	.31**	.24**	–												7.41 (3.51)
8. Phone-C	.10	.16	.04	–.04	.12	.41**	.68**	–											7.09 (3.84)
9. Visits-M	–.10	.09	–.14	–.03	.08	.17	.27**	.16	–										3.20 (3.63)
10. Visits-C	–.02	.20*	–.07	.10	–.08	.11	.27**	.30**	.74**	–									4.49 (3.93)
11. Visits-CH[f]	.18*	.011	–.02	.15	.08	–.10	.20*	.17	.28**	.27**	–								0.07 (0.26)
12. CBCL-IntM[g]	.13	.09	–.10	.04	.04	.05	.03	–.06	.32**	.17	.07	–							6.91 (6.47)
13. CBCL-IntC	.11	.06	–.22**	.04	–.08	–.08	–.11	–.18*	.09	–.03	.06	.37**	–						7.37 (7.15)
14. CDI[h]	–.14	.05	–.10	.02	–.10	.06	–.04	.02	.11	.04	.07	.23**	.16	–					8.04 (7.07)
15. MASC[i]	–.13	.23**	–.04	.08	–.18**	.09	–.05	.09	–.04	.05	–.01	.17	.14	.40**	–				50.43 (17.97)
16. CBCL-ExtM[j]	–.02	–.06	–.18*	.07	–.02	–.06	.06	–.05	.12	.03	.11	.62**	.23**	.28**	–.02	–			9.91 (9.44)
17. CBCL-ExtC	.06	–.08	–.23**	.10	.05	–.01	.03	–.07	.05	–.10	.09	.29**	.59**	.22**	.07	.52**	–		11.46 (10.44)
18. RBP[k]	.17*	–.05	–.08	–.12	–.10	–.03	.02	.12	–.01	–.04	.12	.20*	.23**	.19*	.04	.28**	.27**	–	4.35 (4.10)
19. Bullying[l]	.06	–.05	–.01	–.28**	–.07	–.01	.12	.18*	–.01	–.00	–.01	.14	.13	.28**	.03	.25**	.15	.54**	6.21 (2.84)

Note: *$p < .05$, **$p < .01$

[a] Child gender was coded as 1 = female, 0 = male
[b] Child ethnicity was coded as 1 = Black, 0 = Not Black
[c] SES was calculated based on mother and caregiver report of occupation and education via the Hollingshead method
[d] M = mother reported variable
[e] C = caregiver reported variable
[f] CH = child-reported variable
[g] CBCL-Int = Child Behavior Checklist-Internalizing Behavior Subscale
[h] CDI = child depression inventory
[i] MASC = multidimensional anxiety scale for children
[j] CBCL-Ext = Child Behavior Checklist-Externalizing Behavior Subscale
[k] RBP = risky behavior protocol
[l] Bullying = kids in my class at school

Table 2.2 Mother and caregiver reports of child's contact with the incarcerated mother

Reporter	Mothers	Caregivers	Correlation	t-Value (df)
Mode of contact				
Frequency of phone contact	7.41 (3.51)	7.09 (3.84)	.68**	2.38 (120)*
Frequency of mail contact	5.57 (3.76)	5.88 (3.68)	.39**	1.00 (119)
Frequency of visitation	3.20 (3.62)	4.49 (3.93)	.74**	4.84 (123)**

Note: *p<.05, **p<.01

Crawfordville, FL). Covariance matrices were analyzed using full-information maximum likelihood estimation (FIML[3]). To test our hypotheses, Visits and Alternative Forms of Contact (letters and telephone calls) (as well as lack of contact, see Hypothesis 2) were modeled as simultaneous predictors of internalizing and externalizing behaviors. Residual error terms for observed variables reported by the same reporter (e.g., e1, e3, e5, e9, and e13 in the case of mother-reported variables) were specified to be intercorrelated (these paths are omitted from Fig. 2.1 for clarity of presentation). Child age, gender, ethnicity, and SES were controlled by specifying these variables as exogenous predictors of both outcome variables.

Hypothesis 1: Comparisons of Global vs. Differentiated Contact Models. Our first hypothesis concerned the utility of conceptualizing children's contact with their incarcerated mothers as a global or discrete construct and we hypothesized that a model differentiating visits from phone calls and letters would fit the data better than a model depicting contact as a singular construct. Using mothers' and caregivers' reports of phone calls and letters and mothers', caregivers' and children's reports of frequency of visits, we examined the fit of a global model of "contact". This model (not shown) attempted to have all contact variables load onto a single latent "General Contact" variable. This model did not evidence good fit, X^2 (28)=126.47, $p=.00$; NFI=.61; CFI=.62; RMSEA=.16 (RMSEA 95 % CI=.13–.18). Instead, the second model (shown in the left half of Fig. 2.1) with a latent visits and a latent second-order alternative contact variable (comprised telephone calls and letters) evidenced excellent fit, X^2 (17)=27.59, $p=.50$; NFI=.91; CFI=.96; RMSEA=.06 (RMSEA 95 % CI=.00–.10).

Hypothesis 2: Differences in Visits versus Phone Calls and Letters. The model presented in Fig. 2.1 was tested using SEM. Fit indexes indicated adequate fit, X^2 (92)=135.2, $p=.00$; NFI=.83; CFI=.93; RMSEA=.06 (RMSEA 95 % CI=.04–.08). Standardized and unstandardized parameter estimates appear in Table 2.3 and Fig. 2.1 (paths significant at the $p<.05$ level are in bold). Visits predicted internalizing ($\beta=.27, p=.03$) but not externalizing ($\beta=-.09$, ns) behavior problems. Alternative forms of contact (i.e., letters, calls) also predicted internalizing ($\beta=-.33$, $p=.01$) but not externalizing ($\beta=-.06$, ns) behavior problems.

---

[3] FIML was used to account for missing data. Data were missing at random. Less than 3 % of children and less than 9 % of mothers had missing data across all measures with all caregivers having complete protocols. Incomplete child data were generally due to fatigue whereas for mothers, missing data resulted when they had another activity scheduled at the facility (e.g., lunch) that interfered with finishing the interview or they were transferred to another facility.

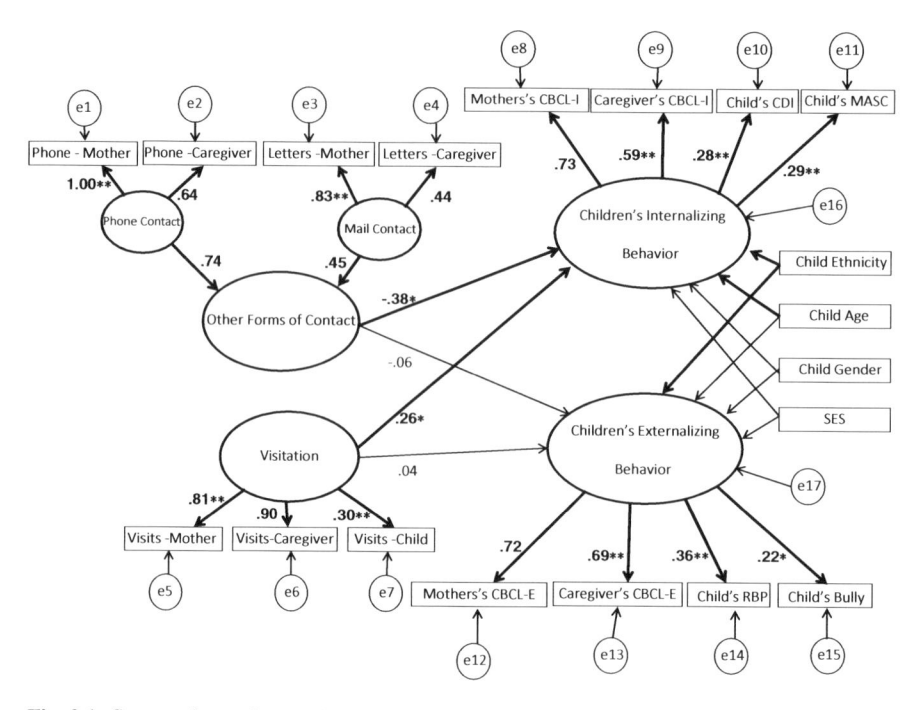

Fig. 2.1 Structural equation model testing the impact of different forms of contact in children's internalizing and externalizing behavior among children with incarcerated mothers (N=147 Children-Mother-Caregiver Triads). Note: *CBCL-I* Child Behavior Checklist-Internalizing Behavior Problems Subscale, *CDI* Children's Depression Inventory, *MASC* Multidimensional Anxiety Scale for Children, *CBCL-E* Child Behavior Checklist Externalizing Behavior Problems Subscale, *RBP* Risky Behavior Protocol, *Bully* Kids in my Class at School. Child Ethnicity was dichotomized as 1=Black, 0=Not Black and Child Gender was dichotomized as 1=female, 0=male. In the model tested, error terms for variables assessed by same participant were correlated

Of note, these effects were in opposite directions; that is, more frequent barrier visitation was associated with more symptoms of internalizing behavior, whereas more phone calls and letters were associated with fewer symptoms of internalizing behavior.

Hypothesis 3: Impact of No or Lack of Contact. Lastly, we examined the associations between lack of contact on children's internalizing and externalizing behaviors. There was only a small number of children who were not in contact with their mothers ($n=26$, 17.7 %, $n=15$ boys). Using independent samples t-tests, we compared children with no contact to children in contact with their incarcerated mothers on key variables (i.e., CBCL, SES). These results are presented in Table 2.4. There were no significant differences between children who had no contact with their incarcerated mothers and children who had some type of contact with their incarcerated mothers on most study variables. However, children's self-report of risky behavior and bullying differed significantly in these two groups such that those who were in contact with their incarcerated mother reported more of these behaviors. Follow-up regression analyses indicated that the difference in children's self-reported risky behavior remained significant when child's age, gender, ethnicity and SES were controlled for ($\beta = .07$, $\Delta r2 = .03$).

Table 2.3 Unstandardized, standardized, and significance levels for model in Fig. 2.1 (standard errors in parentheses, N = 147)

Parameter estimate	Unstandardized	Standardized	p
Measurement model estimates			
Child age → children's internalizing behavior	0.06 (0.02)	.249	.01
Child age → children's externalizing behavior	0.02 (0.03)	.063	.52
Child gender[a] → children's internalizing behavior	1.86 (1.03)	.189	.07
Child gender → children's externalizing behavior	−1.11 (1.42)	−.078	.43
Child ethnicity[b] → children's internalizing behavior	−2.47 (1.09)	−.249	.02
Child ethnicity → children's externalizing behavior	−4.28 (1.50)	−.296	.00
SES[c] → children's internalizing behavior	0.30 (0.59)	.052	.61
SES → children's externalizing behavior	0.63 (0.85)	.075	.46
Children's internalizing behavior → mother's CBCL-I[d]	1.00 (−)	.731	−
Children's internalizing behavior → caregiver's CBCL-I	0.87 (0.18)	.585	.00
Children's internalizing behavior → child's CDI[e]	0.41 (0.14)	.283	.01
Children's internalizing behavior → child's MASC[f]	1.08 (0.38)	.292	.01
Children's externalizing behavior → mother's CBCL-E[g]	1.00 (−)	.720	−
Children's externalizing behavior → caregiver's CBCL-E	1.01 (0.21)	.694	.00
Children's externalizing behavior → child's RBP[h]	0.21 (0.06)	.361	.00
Children's externalizing behavior → child's bullying[i]	0.09 (0.04)	.223	.03
Letters → letter-M[j]	1.91 (0.73)	.827	.01
Letters → letters-C[k]	1.00 (−)	.435	−
Phone → phone-M	1.51 (0.44)	1.00	.00
Phone → phone-C	1.00 (−)	.641	−
Letters → alternative contact	0.93 (1.19)	.449	.43
Phone → alternative contact	1.00 (−)	.738	−
Visits → visits-M	0.84 (0.16)	.811	.00
Visits → visits-C	1.00 (−)	.899	−
Visits → visits-Ch[l]	0.02 (0.01)	.295	.00
Structural model			
Alternative contact → children's internalizing behavior	−0.56 (0.27)	−.382	.04
Alternative contact → children's externalizing behavior	−0.13 (0.25)	−.061	.60
Visits → children's internalizing behavior	0.37 (0.19)	.264	.05
Visits → children's externalizing behavior	0.09 (0.23)	.041	.72

(continued)

Table 2.3 (continued)

Parameter estimate	Unstandardized	Standardized	p
Visits → letters	−0.05 (0.64)	−.009	.94
Visits → phone	2.67 (1.08)	.311	.01
Letters → phone	1.52 (0.765)	.384	.04
e16 → e17	18.14 (5.88)	.658	.00

Note: X^2 (91) = 135.2, p = .00; NFI = .83; CFI = .93; RMSEA = .06 (RMSEA 95 % CI = .04–.08)
[a]*Child Gender* was scored as 1 = Female 0 = male
[b]*Child ethnicity* was dichotomized as 1 = Black, 0 = Not Black
[c]*SES* = Socioeconomic status derived from Hollingshead Index
[d]*CBCL-I* = Child Behavior Checklist-Internalizing Behavior Problems Subscale
[e]*CDI* = children's depression inventory
[f]*MASC* = multidimensional anxiety scale for children
[g]*CBCL-E* = Child Behavior Checklist-Externalizing Behavior Problems Subscale
[h]*RBP* = risky behavior protocol
[i]*Bullying* = kids in my class at school
[j]M = mother reported variable
[k]C = caregiver reported variable
[l]CH = child-reported variable

Table 2.4 Children's psychological outcomes as a function of their lack of contact with an incarcerated mother

	Child is in contact with their incarcerated mother (n = 119)	Caregivers report that child is not in contact with incarcerated mother (n = 26)	t-Value	Cohen's d
Demographic variables				
Child age	119.11 (19.82)	114.54 (20.89)	1.05	.18
Child gender	0.47 (0.50)	0.42 (0.50)	0.44	.07
Child ethnicity	0.60 (0.49)	0.69 (0.47)	0.90	.15
SES	1.83 (0.85)	1.77 (0.86)	0.31	.05
Psychological outcome variables				
Mother's CBCL-I	7.16 (6.87)	6.13 (4.57)	0.70	.12
Caregiver's CBCL-I	7.17 (7.08)	8.73 (7.63)	1.00	.17
Child CDI	8.15 (6.59)	8.00 (9.05)	0.96	.16
Child MASC	51.01 (17.06)	51.02 (21.41)	0.00	.00
Mother's CBCL-E	9.95 (9.92)	9.71 (6.75)	0.11	.02
Caregiver's CBCL-E	11.26 (10.60)	12.38 (9.86)	0.50	.08
Child's RBP	4.65 (4.29)	2.96 (2.52)	1.93*	.32
Child's report of Bullying	6.47 (2.90)	5.28 (2.19)	1.94*	.33

Note: *p < .05
Child Gender was scored as 1 = Female 0 = male. *Child ethnicity* was dichotomized as 1 = Black, 0 = Not Black. *SES* Socioeconomic status derived from Hollingshead Index, *CBCL-I* Child Behavior Checklist-Internalizing Behavior Problems Subscale, *CDI* children's depression inventory, *MASC* multidimensional anxiety scale for children, *CBCL-E* Child Behavior Checklist-Externalizing Behavior Problems Subscale, *RBP* risky behavior protocol, *Bullying* kids in my class at school

2.4 Discussion

The overarching goal of this study was to examine what type of contact, if any, best attends to the unique psychological needs of middle childhood age children who are separated from their mothers because of incarceration in jail. The results point to the importance of examining the type of contact that children have with their incarcerated mothers rather than considering all types of contact as one global construct. Importantly, frequency of children's visits and alternative forms of contact with their incarcerated mothers was related differently to internalizing and externalizing behavior problems. Specifically, children who experienced more frequent barrier visits with their mothers in the jail setting exhibited more self- and other-reported depression and anxiety symptoms, whereas the use of alternative forms of contact (mail, phone) was associated with fewer symptoms of internalizing behavior. Children may be able to create their own gentler version of reality about their incarcerated mother that is abruptly dispelled when they encounter an in-person visit that is compounded by the barrier of Plexiglass. The visit may evoke feelings of worry and sadness that may be suppressed when in the safety of their home and perhaps assuaged when receiving more distant forms of communication. Although the literature indicates that children of incarcerated parents often experience elevated externalizing behavior problems (Murray et al., 2012), in the current study type of contact was not associated with externalizing behavior problems. However, given that between 25 and 29 % of the participants in the current study scored at or above the clinical range for externalizing behaviors, these children likely may have elevated levels of externalizing behaviors compared to other children. These results are thought provoking, particularly with respect to the implications for developing best practices for mother-child contact while mothers are incarcerated in jail settings. However, there are several points that must be considered and evaluated further with additional research before definitive conclusions can be reached.

The quality of phone calls and letters and particularly visits was not assessed but is an important aspect of contact that must be considered when examining the benefits and detriments of different types of contact with incarcerated parents (Folk, Nichols, Dallaire, & Loper, 2012). For example, some of the negative sequelae of visits with incarcerated mothers found in this study may have resulted from visits occurring with Plexiglas window barriers, with mothers dressed in prison garb. Children may be concerned or confused when they are not allowed to touch their incarcerated parents. Such factors may diminish the experience of a visit for children in the 7–12 age range.

Another important factor to consider is the frequency of maternal incarcerations and the degree of associated disruption to the child's life. Certain types of contact may help children cope with change if they have experienced multiple upheavals in their lives due to recurring maternal and/or paternal incarcerations. Further, the stability of the caregiver in children's lives also plays an important role, as well as their support or discouragement of contact with the incarcerated mother.

Although visitation was related to more internalizing symptoms in this study, the directionality of effects could not be determined with the cross-sectional design. Perhaps children who have more internalizing symptoms seek more visits with their incarcerated mothers, whereas children with fewer internalizing symptoms may find letter writing and phone contact to be sufficiently satisfying as a means of staying in contact with their mothers. It was interesting that neither visits nor phone calls and letters was related to externalizing behaviors. It may be that contact reminds children of their feelings of loss associated with their mother's absence because the mother-child separation continues following the visit. These internalizing, sadness-evoking responses may either be intensified by visits or lessened by letters and phone calls but do not appear to be associated with angry, acting-out types of responses. The current study adds to the growing literature in this field which demonstrates the usefulness of an attachment framework when approaching and addressing questions related to the impact of maternal incarceration on children's well-being (e.g., Dallaire et al., 2010; Poehlmann, 2005).

We were surprised that children who had no contact with their incarcerated mothers did not evidence greater internalizing or externalizing behavior problems. To the contrary, children in contact with their incarcerated mother self-reported greater risky behaviors than children who were not in contact with their incarcerated mother. This finding highlights the need to better understand processes that underlie contact. Children who are more risk aversive may avoid being in contact with their incarcerated mother or perhaps the caregiver limits the child's ability to be in contact with his or her mother. This result should be interpreted cautiously and carefully for several reasons. First, the sample size available for this analysis was quite small and thus, these analyses may be under-powered and these findings need to be replicated with larger samples. Second, mothers in the sample were recruited specifically because they could provide valid contact information for the children's caregiver and because they maintained their parental rights. It is possible that children whose mothers are no longer involved in their lives evidence more problematic outcomes but were not sampled in this study. Both of these possibilities should be examined in future research.

The findings and shortcomings of this research suggest several avenues for future research. First, our findings are only generalizable to families in which there was some evidence of connection between the incarcerated mother and person caring for the child. Children's contact and lack of contact with an incarcerated mother and impact on children's mental health, may be very different in families in which the mother is estranged from the child and child's caregiver. Qualitative and narrative data would enrich our understanding of these processes and understanding of how children feel and behave when they get letters, phone calls and visit with their incarcerated mothers. Previous research (e.g., Folk et al., 2012) suggests that the emotional content of the interaction impacts the child's response to the contact. More in-depth analysis of the interaction quality and emotional tone is needed in future research. For example, children who visit a depressed mother may leave that visitation experience feeling depressed. Additional child factors should be examined as well, particularly with regard to children's developmental status. Herein we examined children between the ages of 7 and 12. It is unclear if the same pattern of results would be obtained using a sample of younger children or adolescents. Maternal and caregiver characteristics (e.g., mental health) could also impact amount of contact and should be examined in future research.

In conclusion, these findings have practical implications for families who wish to remain in contact with their incarcerated loved ones via phone, letters and visits. Our data suggest that maintaining regular contact with an incarcerated mother via phone calls and letters may help children continue to feel connected to her and allay feelings of depression and anxiety. The results of the current study also add to the growing body of literature suggesting that non-contact visitation experiences that occur through a Plexiglas barrier may be associated with more problematic outcomes in this population. Families can help prepare children for a visit with their incarcerated loved one by letting them know the rules for visitation at the facility and what to expect when they arrive, as well as help the children process the visit and emotions the child may be having after the visit.

Acknowledgements This research was funded by grant # 5R21HD060104-02 to the College of William & Mary and the first two authors by the National Institutes of Health. The authors would also like to thank the many students and collaborators who made this research possible, including Caroline Cumings, Johanna Folk, Jennifer Poon, Adrian Bravo and Jasmine Hedge.

References

Achenbach, T. M., & Rescorla, L. A. (2001). *Manual for the ASEBA school-age forms & profiles.* Burlington, VT: University of Vermont, Research Center for Children, Youth, and Families.

Arditti, J. A., Lambert-Shute, J., & Joest, K. (2003). Saturday morning at the jail: Implications of incarceration for families and children. *Family Relations: An Interdisciplinary Journal of Applied Family Studies, 52*(3), 195–204. doi:10.1111/j.1741-3729.2003.00195.x.

Baldwin, J. S., & Dadds, M. R. (2007). Reliability and validity of parent and child versions of the multidimensional anxiety scale for children in community samples. *Journal of the American Academy of Child and Adolescent Psychiatry, 46*(2), 252–260. doi:10.1097/01.chi.0000246065.93200.a1.

Bales, W. D., & Mears, D. P. (2008). Inmate social ties and the transition to society: Does visitation reduce recidivism? *Journal of Research in Crime and Delinquency, 45*(3), 287–321. doi:10.1177/0022427808317574.

Brumariu, L. E., & Kerns, K. A. (2010). Parent-child attachment and internalizing symptoms in childhood and adolescence: A review of empirical findings and future directions. *Development and Psychopathology, 22*(1), 177–203. doi:10.1017/S0954579409990344.

Carey, M. P., Gresham, F. M., Ruggiero, L., Faulstich, M. E., & Enyart, P. (1987). Children's depression inventory: Construct and discriminant validity across clinical and nonreferred (control) populations. *Journal of Consulting and Clinical Psychology, 55*(5), 755–761. doi:10.1037/0022-006X.55.5.755.

Conger, R. D., Elder, G. H., Jr., Lorenz, F. O., Simons, R. L., & Whitbeck, L. B. (1994). *Families in troubled times: Adapting to change in rural America.* Hawthorne, NY: Aldine de Gruyter.

Dallaire, D. H., Zeman, J. L., & Thrash, T. (2015). Children's experiences of maternal incarceration-specific risks: Predictions to psychological maladaptation. *Journal of Clinical Child and Adolescent Psychology, 44,* 109–122.

Dallaire, D. H. (2007). Incarcerated mothers and fathers: A comparison of risks for children and families. *Family Relations, 56*(5), 440–453. doi:10.1111/j.1741-3729.2007.00472.x.

Dallaire, D. H., Ciccone, A., & Wilson, L. (2010). Teachers' experiences with and expectations of children with incarcerated parents. *Journal of Applied Developmental Psychology, 31*(4), 281–290. doi:10.1016/j.appdev.2010.04.001.

Dallaire, D. H., Ciccone, A., & Wilson, L. (2012). The family drawings of at-risk children: Concurrent relations with contact with incarcerated parents, caregiver behavior and stress. *Attachment & Human Development, 14*(2), 161–183. doi:10.1080/14616734.2012.661232.

Deonandan, R., Campbell, M. K., Ostbye, T., Tummon, I., & Robertson, J. (2001). IVF births and pregnancies: An exploration of two methods of assessment using life-table analysis. *Journal of Assisted Reproduction and Genetics, 18*(2), 73–77. doi:10.1023/A:1026526523666.

Folk, J. B., Nichols, E. B., Dallaire, D. H., & Loper, A. B. (2012). Evaluating the content and reception of messages from incarcerated parents to their children. *American Journal of Orthopsychiatry, 82*(4), 529–541. doi:10.1111/j.1939-0025.2012.01179.x.

Hollingshead, A. B. (1957). *Two factor index of social position*. New Haven, CT: Yale University.

Kazdin, A. E. (1989). Identifying depression in children: A comparison of alternative selection criteria. *Journal of Abnormal Child Psychology, 17*(4), 437–454. doi:10.1007/BF00915037.

Kovacs, M. (1992). *Children's depression inventory: Manual*. North Tonawanda, NY: Multi-Health Systems.

Ladd, G. W., Kochenderfer, B. J., & Coleman, C. (1996). Friendship quality as a predictor of young children's early school adjustment. *Child Development, 67*(3), 1103–1118. doi:10.2307/1131882.

Ladd, G. W., Kochenderfer, B. J., & Coleman, C. (1997). Classroom peer acceptance, friendship and victimization: Distinct relational systems that contribute uniquely to children's school adjustment? *Child Development, 68*(6), 1181–1197. doi:10.2307/1132300.

Lilenfeld, S. O. (2003). Comorbidity between and within childhood externalizing and internalizing disorders: Reflections and directions. *Journal of Abnormal Child Psychology, 31*, 285–291. doi:10.1023/A:1023229529866.

March, J. S. (1997). *Multidimensional anxiety scale for children: Technical manual*. North Tonawanda, NY: Multi-Health Systems.

Maruschak, L. M., Glaze, L. E., & Mumola, C. J. (2010). Incarcerated parents and their children. In J. M. Eddy & J. Poehlmann (Eds.), *Children of incarcerated parents: A handbook for researchers and practitioners* (pp. 33–51). Washington, DC: Urban Institute Press.

Murray, J., Farrington, D. P., & Sekol, I. (2012). Children's antisocial behavior, mental health, drug use, and educational performance after parental incarceration: A systematic review and meta-analysis. *Psychological Bulletin, 138*(2), 175–210. doi:10.1037/a0026407.

Perdue, N. H., Manzeske, D. P., & Estell, D. B. (2009). Early predictors of school engagement: Exploring the role of peer relationships. *Psychology in the Schools, 46*(10), 1084–1097. doi:10.1002/pits.20446.

Poehlmann, J. (2005). Representations of attachment relationships in children of incarcerated mothers. *Child Development, 76*, 679–696.

Poehlmann, J., Dallaire, D. H., Loper, A. B., & Shear, L. D. (2010). Children's contact with their incarcerated parents: Research findings and recommendations. *American Psychologist, 65*(6), 575–598. doi:10.1037/a0020279.

Poehlmann, J., & Eddy, M. J. (2013). Relationship processes and resilience in children with incarcerated parents. *Monographs of the Society for Research in Child Development, 78*, 1–6.

Purvis, M. (2013). Paternal incarceration and parenting programs in prison: A review paper. *Psychiatry Psychology and Law, 20*, 9–28.

Rudasill, K. M., Reio, T. G., Jr., Stipanovic, N., & Taylor, J. E. (2010). A longitudinal study of student-teacher relationship quality, difficult temperament, and risky behavior from childhood to early adolescence. *Journal of School Psychology, 48*(5), 389–412. doi:10.1016/j.jsp.2010.05.001.

Shiner, R. L. (1998). How shall we speak of children's personalities in middle childhood? A preliminary taxonomy. *Psychological Bulletin, 124*(3), 308–332. doi:10.1037/0033-2909.124.3.308.

Shlafer, R. J., & Poehlmann, J. (2010). Attachment and caregiving relationships in families affected by parental incarceration. *Attachment & Human Development, 12*(4), 395–415. doi:10.1080/14616730903417052.

Smucker, M. R., Craighead, W. E., Craighead, L. W., & Green, B. J. (1986). Normative and reliability data for the children's depression inventory. *Journal of Abnormal Child Psychology, 14*(1), 25–39. doi:10.1007/BF00917219.

Tuerk, E. H., & Loper, A. B. (2006). Contact between incarcerated mothers and their children: Assessing parenting stress. *Journal of Offender Rehabilitation, 43*(1), 23–43. doi:10.1300/J076v43n01_02.

Zeman, J., Cassano, M., & Adrian, M. (2013). Socialization influences on children's and adolescents' emotional self-regulation processes: A developmental psychopathology perspective. In K. Barrett, G. Morgan, & N. Fox (Eds.), *Handbook of self-regulatory processes in development: New directions and international perspectives* (pp. 79–107). New York: Routledge.

Chapter 3
Young Children's Behavioral and Emotional Reactions to Plexiglas and Video Visits with Jailed Parents

Julie Poehlmann-Tynan, Hilary Runion, Cynthia Burnson, Sarah Maleck, Lindsay Weymouth, Kierra Pettit, and Mary Huser

3.1 Introduction

In the 12-month period ending June 2013, jails across the US admitted an estimated 11.7 million people, similar to the previous year (Minton & Golinelli, 2014). About 47.2 % of jail inmates were White, 35.8 % were Black, and 14.8 % were Latino. National estimates indicate that approximately 86 % of people in jail in 2013 were men; whereas the number of jailed women increased 10.9 % between 2010 and 2013, the number of jailed men declined 4.2 % (Minton & Golinelli, 2014). An earlier national survey found that 36 % of jail inmates had at least one child under 15 years (Kemper & Rivara, 1993). Put together, these surveys suggest that millions of children experience a parent's admission to jail in the US each year. Although the actual numbers are unknown because corrections, schools, and child welfare systems do not systematically collect information about the parental status of incarcerated individuals (Eddy & Poehlmann, 2010), it is clear that parental incarceration has become a major public health concern in the US. If the current estimates are correct, having an incarcerated parent occurs at 3.5 times the rate of autism and twice the rate of child maltreatment.

Children of incarcerated parents are more likely to experience multiple risk factors and develop problematic outcomes than their peers, including substance

---

J. Poehlmann-Tynan, Ph.D. (✉) • H. Runion • C. Burnson • S. Maleck
L. Weymouth • K. Pettit
Human Development & Family Studies, University of Wisconsin-Madison,
Madison, WI, USA
e-mail: poehlmann@waisman.wisc.edu

M. Huser
Cooperative Extension Family Living Programs,
University of Wisconsin-Extension, Madison, WI, USA

abuse, externalizing problems, academic difficulties and school failure, truancy, criminal activity, and persistent anxiety or depression as well as health problems (Center for Disease Control, 2009; Murray & Farrington, 2008; Murray, Farrington, Sekol, & Olsen, 2009). However, many existing studies of children with incarcerated parents have involved secondary analysis of data collected for other purposes, and these studies have typically not included information about children's incarceration-specific experiences such as contact with the incarcerated parent (Murray et al., 2009). Moreover, previous studies have often combined prison and jail samples—indeed, the term "parental incarceration" is an umbrella term that refers to parents in prison or jail (Poehlmann & Eddy, 2013). However, prison and jail populations may differ in systematic ways, such as crime severity and length of time spent in the corrections facility, and parental prison and jail stays may have different effects on children. Jails and prisons differ as well, with jails being locally operated and prisons, state or federally operated. They also vary in programs offered, type of visitation available to family members, and levels of security. For example, jails are more likely to offer Plexiglas barrier visitation whereas prisons are more likely to offer face-to-face non-barrier visitation (Poehlmann, Dallaire, Loper, & Shear, 2010; Shlafer, Loper, & Schillmoeller, 2015). Despite these differences, few studies have focused on children of jailed parents, and no studies have relied on direct assessment of children with parents in jail. Yet most felons who spend time in prison have a history of jail time (Glaze & Maruschak, 2008), and identifying children during a parent's jail stay may be catching some families early in the process that may eventually result in a parent's longer-term incarceration.

Supportive family relationships and interactions are important for facilitating resilience processes in children with jailed and imprisoned parents (Poehlmann & Eddy, 2013). Although parent–child visits during parental incarceration are one contributing factor to parent–child relationships and individual well-being (Poehlmann et al., 2010), prior studies have not examined the quality of children's visits with incarcerated parents. Less than half of parents in prison report receiving visits from their children (Glaze & Maruschak, 2008), yet it appears to be more common for jailed parents to receive visits from children than imprisoned parents, as jails are locally-operated and located closer to families of inmates than are state or Federal prisons (Arditti, 2012; Arditti, Lambert-Shute, & Joest, 2003).

Some scholars have noted concerns about children visiting jailed parents through Plexiglas barriers because children cannot touch their parents and they can only hear and talk to them through a hand-held telephone device or hole in the barrier (e.g., Arditti et al., 2003). Moreover, concerns have been noted regarding children's experiences of potentially stressful security procedures such as frisking or use of metal detectors (e.g., Dallaire, Ciccone, & Wilson, 2012; Poehlmann et al., 2010). Some prisoner and family advocates have attempted to allay these concerns, in some cases arguing that all children with incarcerated parents have a right to "speak with, see and touch my parent" regardless of the circumstances (San Francisco Children of Incarcerated Parents Partnership, 2005). For example, in one of their fact sheets about children with incarcerated parents, the Osborne Association (2012) states that "visits with parents (in most cases) help to heal the pain of the loss and are critical to children's well-being," although no supporting research is cited. Yet to make such arguments and recommendations without child-focused data is premature; additional data are needed, including examination of children's experiences of and reactions to visitation when their parents are in jail or prison.

Previous studies examining children's contact with their incarcerated parents have focused on frequency of visitation, type of visitation (e.g., face-to-face or barrier visits), and other forms of contact that occur during the incarceration period in comparison to visits (e.g., telephone calls or mail contact versus visits) (see Poehlmann et al., 2010, for a summary). Although frequency and type of visits are important variables to consider when examining family relationships and adjustment of children with incarcerated parents, it is also critical to understand children's experiences visiting corrections facilities and the process of how children relate to their incarcerated parents and caregivers during visitation. Child-focused observational data collected within corrections settings during visitation can help clarify concerns as well as identify strengths of the visitation process for children. Although qualitative data have focused on adult family members' experiences visiting in jail settings (Arditti et al., 2003), quantitative and qualitative approaches have not focused on documenting children's experiences of visitation. Such data can help inform recommendations for what children need during visits with incarcerated parents, including appropriate policies, procedures, and programs for children with jailed parents.

The present report is part of a larger study focusing on young children with jailed parents. As part of the research, ratings of children's behavioral and emotional reactions during visits with jailed parents were recorded. Researchers observed children visiting their jailed parents at three jail sites: one that relied on video visitation, one that used Plexiglas barrier visits, and another that offered both options. Children's affective and behavioral reactions were rated by trained research personnel during security procedures, wait time, and the visit; global ratings were also made regarding children's activity level, behavioral regulation, and emotional regulation during visits to the jail and at home. Although we also collected data focusing on children's attachment relationships, home environments, behavior problems, and cognitive functioning, as well as a myriad of variables reflecting caregivers' and incarcerated parents' well-being, here we focus on our observational data of children's visits to the jail.

Our primary goals for this mixed method study were to describe children's experience of visits with their incarcerated parents in jail settings and to compare children's reactions to video and Plexiglas visits with jailed parents. A secondary goal was to determine if ratings of children's self-regulation and activity level differed in the jail visit setting compared to the home environment. A case study is presented to illustrate a typical video visit between a child and parent, based on our observations. Names and other identifying information were changed to protect confidentiality.

3.2 Method

3.2.1 Participants

Forty-eight children and their caregivers and jailed parents were enrolled in an ongoing study at the time of this report; this report focuses on 20 children who were observed visiting their jailed parents. The families of the 20 (42 %) children observed during visits did not differ from the families of the 28 (58 %) children not observed during visits with respect to caregiver education, family income, months of public assistance received, number of dependents, target child age, and length of time the caregiver was in a relationship with their current partner.

Recruitment efforts began with the jailed parent. Weekly, administrative staff at jails in three Wisconsin counties that represented diverse urban and rural populations provided either the names of newly sentenced parents who had children between 2 and 6 years of age or access to the database with this information. Identified inmates then participated in a brief initial screening with a trained researcher to determine if they met the research criteria indicating that they: (1) were at least 18 years old, (2) had a child who lived with kin within the county in which the inmate was serving time (or an adjacent county), (3) had retained legal rights to the child and had not committed a crime against the child, (4) had cared for the child at least part of the time prior to incarceration, (5) could understand and read English, and (6) had already been sentenced to serve jail time or were accused of committing a crime that would result in jail time (usually a misdemeanor rather than a felony which would result in a lengthier prison sentence). If the inmate had more than one child in the age range, a child was randomly selected for participation in the study. Inmates who met criteria were invited to participate in the study, and those who agreed signed informed consent forms and participated in an interview, vocabulary assessment, and self-administered questionnaires. The study was approved by the Institutional Review Board of the University of Wisconsin and an NIH Certificate of Confidentiality was used.

Three jails participated in this research. The first jail is located in a large urban community that experiences some racial disparities in arrest and incarceration rates. Although 86 % of people in the county are white, approximately half of the jail inmates are African American; for example, of the total 9,276 inmates who spent time in the county jail in 2012, 47 % were Black. The facility has an 823-bed capacity, with an average daily population of 788 inmates (21 % women and 79 % men). In this jail, visits occur through a Plexiglas barrier in a secure section of the jail or through video visitation in a non-secure section of the jail. The second jail site is located in a rural county. The jail has a 458-bed capacity and in 2009, the jail had a daily count of 277 inmates (90 % men, 10 % women), although the daily count declined during the study period. At this jail, visits occur through closed circuit TV in a non-secure part of the jail. The third jail system is located in an urban community and holds a mix of individuals from urban and rural locations. In 2010, the average daily population of the three facilities in this county was 704, although our study focused on only two of the facilities. Visits in these two facilities occur through a Plexiglas barrier in a secure section of the jail.

Characteristics of Children and Families. Of the 20 children observed visiting their jailed parents, children ranged in age from 2 to 6 years, with an average of 3.9 years ($SD = 1.4$). Eleven children were girls and nine were boys. Eighteen children had incarcerated fathers and two children had incarcerated mothers; 80 % of children lived with the non-incarcerated parent and 20 % lived with grandparents. Prior to the current incarceration, most children (80 %) lived with their jailed parents. Jailed parents were incarcerated for drug-related crimes (40 %), probation violations (25 %), nonpayment of child support (15 %), multiple crimes (15 %), and other (5 %). The majority of parents (95 %) were repeat offenders and 80 % had spent time in jail previously. Forty percent of jailed parents were African American, 40 % were Caucasian, 5 % were Latino, and 15 % were multiracial. Families lived between 0.4 and 40 miles from the jail. Incarcerated parents reported varying levels of contact with their children and children's caregivers: 65 % had telephone contact with the child and 70 % had telephone contact with the child's caregiver; 45 % wrote to the child and 50 % wrote to the child's caregiver; and 50 % reported that their child wrote to them while 55 % of caregivers wrote to them. Table 3.1 shows additional demographic characteristics of incarcerated parents and children's caregivers.

Table 3.1 Participant characteristics

Caregivers ($N=20$)	(n, %)	Range
Age (years)		18–62
Gender		
Female	19, 95	
Male	1, 5	
Education		
Partial high school	4, 20	
High school graduate/GED	8, 40	
Partial college	8, 40	
Marital status		
Never married	14, 70	
Currently married	2, 10	
Legally separated	1, 5	
Divorced	2, 10	
Widowed	1, 5	
Employment		
Currently employed	9, 45	
Currently unemployed	11, 55	
Income		
No annual income	3, 15	
($1,200–$7,500)	2, 10	

(continued)

Table 3.1 (continued)

Caregivers (N=20)	(n, %)	Range
($7,600–$14,000)	8, 40	
($14,000–$26,000)	5, 25	
(above $26,000)	2, 10	
Incarcerated parents (N=20)	(n, %)	Range
Age (years)		18–46
Gender		
Female	2, 10	
Male	18, 90	
Education		
Partial high school	4, 20	
High school/GED	7, 35	
Partial college	9, 45	
Marital status		
Never married	14, 70	
Currently married	2, 10	
Legally separated	1, 5	
Divorced	3, 15	
Length of sentence (days)		Unknown–1,095
Unknown	7, 35	
30–60	5, 25	
61–119	2, 10	
120 days and over	6, 30	
Amount of time served (days)		7–120
0–14	7, 35	
15–30	4, 20	
31–59	5, 25	
60–120	4, 20	

3.2.2 Procedure

Consented inmates were interviewed by a researcher in a private area within the cell block, with security staff nearby. We asked jailed parents about demographics, children's living arrangements prior to and following incarceration (i.e., caregiving stability), children's experience of incarcerated-related events (e.g., distress resulting from witnessing the parent's crime, arrest, sentencing), and previous and current contact with children and children's caregivers. During interviews with jailed parents, researchers also asked the inmate: for the contact information of the child's caregiver; to sign a consent form for the child's participation and for the observed jail visit; and to sign release forms to contact the child's caregiver. We were unable to compensate jailed parents for their study participation.

Researchers contacted children's caregivers by phone, letter, in person, email or text messages. Children and caregivers were assessed in two settings: a visit with the jailed parent and a home visit. During the initial visit, caregivers were asked to sign an informed consent form for their own and the child's participation (read aloud because of potential literacy issues), and children were asked for verbal assent.

Jail visit. During the jail data collection, which lasted between 20 and 90 min (depending on the wait time and length of visit), the child's visit with the jailed parent was observed and rated. Children were accompanied to the jail visit by their caregivers. A researcher met the family at the entrance to the jail and observed the child during security procedures, wait time, and during the visit with the jailed parent. Visits occurred either through closed circuit television (i.e., video visit) or through Plexiglas (i.e., barrier visit). In both types of visits, the caregiver and child (and observer) could see the jailed parent from a booth. However, only one family member at a time could speak with and hear the jailed parent through a headset similar to a telephone receiver. The observer was not able to hear or interact with the jailed parent, although the jailed parent knew that the observer was present (and previously had provided written consent for the observation). Observers were able to see and hear the child, and thus they focused on rating the child's emotional and behavioral reactions to the visit rather than adult behaviors. Caregivers were paid $50 following the observed jail visit.

Home visit. Two trained researchers conducted a home visit with the child and caregiver that lasted 2 to 3 h and included interviews, standardized assessments, observations of the home environment, videotaped caregiver-child play interactions, and self-administered questionnaires. One researcher interviewed the caregiver and the other assessed the child. Caregivers were paid $50 following the home visit and children were given an age-appropriate book. In this report, we focused on global ratings of children's behaviors in the home environment to compare with the ratings made in the jail setting.

3.2.3 Measures

The Jail-Prison Observation Checklist (JPOC, Appendix A; Poehlmann, 2012) was used to rate children's reactions to visits. The JPOC is an observational rating scale designed to be rated in vivo by trained researchers in jail or prison settings starting from when a child enters the corrections facility for a visit until the time that the child leaves. Because researchers are generally not able to videotape in corrections setting, ratings are made live, as the behaviors occur, and interrater reliability is established in the corrections setting.

Observers rate the presence or absence of security procedures (metal detector, frisking of adults or children, shoe removal, bag search, and checking identification), and the presence or absence of children's behaviors in the following domains: Child's Affect During Entry, Wait, and Visit; Child's Attachment Behaviors During Entry, Wait, and Visit; and Child's Behaviors Toward the Incarcerated Parent. Additional items refer to cleanliness and noise in the jail or prison environment, families' interactions with staff members, length of wait time, type of visit, length of visit, and presence of child-friendly materials (e.g., stickers, coloring materials). Following the visit, researchers also complete global ratings of children's activity level, behavioral dysregulation (i.e., how well the child is able to modify their own behaviors in response to demands of the context), and emotional lability as displayed throughout their time at the corrections facility. These ratings are made on a 1 to 5 scale, with higher ratings indicating more activity, dysregulation and lability.

For the present study, interrater reliability for items on the JPOC was established between two independent observers across 15 observed jail visits. Intraclass correlation coefficients (ICCs) fell within an acceptable to high range. ICCs for Security Procedures items ranged from .70 to 1.0 with a mean of .93, Child's Affect During Entry ranged from .65 to 1.0, with a mean of .89, and Child's Attachment Behaviors During Entry ranged from .75 to 1.0 with a mean of .93. In addition, Child's Affect During Wait ranged from .55 to 1.0 (mean = .83), Child's Attachment Behavior During Wait range from .80 to 1.0 (mean = .93), Child's Affect During Visit ranged from .65 to .90 (mean = .78), Child's Attachment Behavior During Visit ranged from .85 to 1.0 (mean = .87), and Child's Behavior Towards Incarcerated Parent ranged from .75 to 1.0 (mean = .91). The six items on the Security Procedures scale were summed to reflect total number of security procedures used in the jails (Cronbach's α = .65). ICCs for global ratings of children's behaviors in the jail were .50 for exact ratings but significantly higher when ratings were examined within one point (activity level = .95, behavioral dysregulation = 1.0, and emotional lability = .85). Global ratings of children were also made in the home, at the end of the home visit in which the research team collected data that is summarized in other reports. ICCs for global ratings of children's behaviors in the home ranged from .45 to .70 for exact ratings but were higher when ratings were examined within one point (activity level = 1.0, behavioral dysregulation = 1.0, and emotional lability = .95).

3.3 Results

First we describe the findings from the Jail-Prison Observation Checklist regarding security procedures, children's affect, children's behaviors exhibited toward caregivers and incarcerated parents in the jail setting, and ratings of jail environments. Second, we examine potential differences between ratings of video and Plexiglas visits and between children's behaviors in the jail and home settings. Third, we present themes identified regarding the content of children's visits with incarcerated parents. Finally, we present a case study that illustrates a typical visit that our research team observed (with names and identifying information removed).

Security Procedures. Twelve of the observed visits occurred via closed circuit television (i.e., video visit) and eight visits occurred through a Plexiglas barrier. Three out of four children were accompanied to the jail by their mothers, whereas one-quarter were brought by their grandmothers. One-fourth of children were also

Table 3.2 Security procedures experienced by children and caregivers upon entry to the jail ($n=20$)

Security procedures		Frequency	(%)
Metal detector used?	Yes	6	30
	No	14	70
Adults frisked?	Yes	1	5
	No	19	95
Children frisked?	Yes	0	0
	No	20	100
Shoes removed?	Yes	4	30
	No	16	70
Bags searched?	Yes	5	25
	No	15	75
Check identification?	Yes	17	85
	No	3	15

accompanied by at least one other child, although only the target child was observed and rated. For seven target children (35 %), the observed visit was their first visit to the jail.

Table 3.2 indicates the type of security procedures experienced by children and their caregivers in the jail settings. Most families needed to show some form of identification to enter the jail setting, most often a driver's license for the adult and sometimes a birth certificate for the child. Slightly less than half of children were asked to go through a metal detector, and some families were asked to remove their shoes or present their bag for search. Notably, no children were frisked or patted down at any of the jails.

Children's Affect and Attachment Behaviors. Table 3.3 shows ratings of children's emotional expressions during entry and security procedures, wait time, and the visit, as well as children's attachment behaviors directed toward their caregivers while at the jail. Most children stayed in close proximity to their caregivers for the duration of their time at the jail, and the majority of children engaged in a high level of contact maintenance by the time the visit ended (e.g., sitting on the caregiver's lap, clinging to the caregiver's leg, holding the caregiver's hand). Although no children displayed avoidant or aggressive behavior toward their caregivers during entry and security procedures, by the end of the visit nearly half of children (45 %) engaged in avoidance and 15 % hit or pushed their caregivers. Both contact maintenance and distress appeared to increase the longer that the children were in the corrections facility. Although all children appeared happy at some point during their visit with the incarcerated parent, there was also an increase in negative affective expression between the time that children entered the jail and when they finished their visit, especially fatigue, confusion, sadness, and anger. Only 10 % of children expressed fear. Throughout their time at the jail, most children were observed to alternate between two predominant emotional expressions: happy and serious/somber facial expressions.

Table 3.3 Frequency of children's attachment behaviors towards caregivers and affect during entry, wait, and visit (n=20)

Child's behavior or emotion	Entry	Wait	Visit
Proximity seeking	18	19	17
Hand holding	3	4	4
Clinging	7	11	14
Crying	2	1	1
Whining	3	5	9
Pushing	0	1	3
Avoiding	0	2	9
Hitting	0	1	3
Tired	4	8	13
Confused	5	6	11
Fearful	1	2	2
Sad	2	2	7
Happy	15	16	20
Angry	1	1	6
Serious/Somber	14	15	19
Self-Soothing	6	7	7

Children's Behavior towards Incarcerated Parents. During the visit, children engaged in a wide range of behaviors toward their incarcerated parents. At some point during the visit, all children engaged in visual contact with incarcerated parents, and 95 % of children talked to their parents and listened to what their parents said. Ninety percent of children responded directly to something that the incarcerated parent said or did, and 80 % of the children did or said something loving to the incarcerated parent, such as blowing kisses or saying "I love you." However, 82 % of children also avoided engaging with the jailed parent at some point during the visit.

Table 3.4 shows the common themes that emerged during children's visits with their incarcerated parents. The themes are based on the notes taken by researchers who observed visits and are arranged in the table from most to least frequent. The notes focused on children's verbalizations, behaviors, and interactions with incarcerated parents and caregivers. Themes are presented to help readers gain a better understanding of the content and process of the visits. The most common themes reflected children having prompted and independent conversations with incarcerated parents, often about events in their daily lives. Another common theme was for children to say "I love you" to their jailed parents. The least common themes involved children becoming distressed or disobeying their caregivers. Table 3.4 provides examples for each theme.

The research team also noted several areas of concern that were not on our rating form but that appeared important for children's visitation experiences. Many children were not familiar with the hand-held device that allowed them to listen to their incarcerated parent. The device looks like a telephone receiver, and many families

Table 3.4 Themes regarding children's visits with jailed parents

Theme	Description	Notes taken during observed visit or quote
Prompted conversation	Child is prompted by caregiver to talk to parent, either told to repeat a phrase or given idea for conversation	Caregiver encouraged child to 'say bye to dad'
		Caregiver told child to say certain things and he tried to repeat them
Independent conversation	Child talks to parent freely, comes up with conversation on own	Child showed her new book 'The Kissing Hand' to dad and talked about her Christmas list in detail
		"Hello? Daddy. I need to tell you my Spanish" (with help from grandmother, recited 1–10 in Spanish)
		Parent held up ten fingers and child said "I don't know the big numbers. I going to bilingual class. I'm going to the gym, we played basketball"
"I Love You"	Child says "I love you" to jailed parent	"Hi dad, I love you too"
		"I love you too, I love you too"
Positive nonverbal expressions	Displays positive emotions toward jailed parent, such as excitement, smiling, i.e., wanting to interact	Child blew kisses through phone
		Child smiled and said "Daddy, I want daddy"
		Child sat on caregiver's lap the whole time
Stays near caregiver	Child sits near or on caregiver	Child stayed very close to caregiver, climbed on chair and walked around chair
Restless or moves around room	Child moves around the room or appears restless	Child shook her head, wriggled on the chair, stood on chair, clapped her hands
		Child ran from one end of room to other; threw a penny; screeched, ran, stood on chair
		Child bobbed back and forth on her chair, made smacking noises with her mouth, zipped her coat up and down
Uninterested	Child appears uninterested in talking to the incarcerated parent	Child not interested in video
		Child avoided talking to incarcerated parent
Distressed	Seems upset or distressed	Child threw phone back at caregiver at the sound of dad's voice. Child received verbal feedback from caregiver about his negative behavior while he kicked and screamed
		Child got up off chair and talked to caregiver in a whining voice. Child became distressed and stomped his feet
Disobeys caregiver	Child ignores caregiver's requests, or does not do what is asked of him/her	Child was scolded by caregiver
		Caregiver called child back, child didn't come back

indicated that they only use cell or mobile phones in their homes. Moreover, it was common for children to watch the visits of people sitting adjacent to them in both Plexiglas and video modalities. Sometimes children were exposed to conversations occurring next to them that may not have been appropriate for children, and in some facilities, children could see behind the inmate into their cell block. In addition, our research team noted that video visits often ended abruptly with the screen turning off without any warning to children. Some caregivers attended to the small timer display at the edge of the screen that indicated when the visit was going to end and they cued the children, although this was not common. Some children appeared distressed by the sudden end to the visit (e.g., "where did daddy go?" while becoming teary).

Ratings of Jail Environments. Our research team also rated aspects of the jail environments, including staff treatment of families, wait time, cleanliness of the facility, noise levels, and whether child-friendly materials were available for children's visits (e.g., stickers, books, coloring materials). The majority of interactions with staff were neutral, and only a few interactions were rated as overtly positive or negative. Wait times ranged from 0 to 65 min, with an average of 18 min ($SD=20$), and visits ranged in length from 12 to 45 min (mean=22, $SD=8$). Noise levels were rated as generally moderate to low, and the facilities were mostly rated as clean. None of the facilities had child-friendly materials available in the visiting area, although one jail had books in a separate area where children may have passed through on their way to the visiting area.

Comparisons. We used independent samples t-tests to compare global ratings of children's behavioral self-regulation, activity level, and emotional lability for video and Plexiglas visits. Ratings did not differ between type of jail visit. We also examined number of security procedures, length of wait time, and length of the visit for video and Plexiglas visits using t-tests. Security procedures differed depending on whether the visit was a video or Plexiglas visit. Families participating in video visits experienced fewer security procedures than families experiencing Plexiglas visits, $t(18)=-2.91$, $p<.01$. Although families waited significantly longer for Plexiglas visits compared with video visits, $t(18)=-5.30$, $p<.001$, with an average of 36 versus 5 min of wait time, Plexiglas visits lasted longer than video visits, $t(19)=-2.62$, $p<.05$, with an average of 28-versus 19-min visits.

We also compared our global ratings of children's behaviors made in the jail setting with those made in the home setting using paired samples t-tests. Although children's activity level did not differ across settings, $t(19)=0.0$, $p=1.0$, children exhibited significantly more behavioral dysregulation in the jail setting compared to the home, $t(19)=2.18$, $p<.05$. There was a trend for children to exhibit slightly more emotional lability in the jail compared to the home, $t(19)=1.80$, $p=.09$. Wait time and number of security procedures were not significantly correlated with global child ratings.

Case Study: Five year old Chelsea and her mother, Marley, drove 3 miles to the jail, like they have done every week for the past 6 weeks. They arrived at the jail, entering the non-secure side and showing Marley's identification as part of the screening process so they could visit with Dave, Chelsea's dad. Dave has almost completed his 45 day jail sentence. The visit was conducted through a video monitor in a small room with about 10 monitors and 20 chairs. As Chelsea approached the video monitor, she became very excited and waved furiously exclaiming "Hi daddy!" as she sat in one of the chairs. Marley settled off to the side a few feet away, and concentrated her attention on her cell phone. Dave occasionally blew kisses to Marley and turned around to the other inmates behind him to gauge their reactions, as his side of the video exchange was being conducted in his cell block. Marley did not respond to his affection. In contrast, Chelsea did not lose eye contact with her father. Dave and Chelsea talked in a playful manner and Chelsea responded positively to his communications. They discussed Christmas presents and Chelsea showed him the book that she received from the researchers who were observing from the corner, trying to go unnoticed. The conversation became more somber when Chelsea admitted, "I cry about you." Dave developed tears in his eyes up and said "Why you crying for me? I don't want you crying about me." The crying ended quickly because Chelsea led the conversation elsewhere. She told her father that she had been sick ("I have been coughing") and he inquired more about how she was feeling. At this point in the visit, Marley came closer and asked her daughter for the phone; she had an abrupt conversation with Dave and then handed the phone back to Chelsea, who had been looking at the video monitors on either side of her. The rest of the conversation occurred mostly between Chelsea and her father. He assured her that his sentence was almost complete and at one point Chelsea turned to the researchers in the corner and said "My dad gets out in two days". Throughout the rest of the conversation, Marley occasionally took the phone to bring up custody and family issues with Dave, while Chelsea either watched her dad's face on the monitor or gazed at the other monitors in the room while wiggling in her chair. Towards the end of the visit Chelsea repeatedly looked at her father and said "I love you too, I love you too". The visit abruptly ended when the video screen turned black. Chelsea said "He gone" and looked serious until she left with her mother.

3.4 Discussion

Ratings of visit quality can help inform recommendations for procedures and policies for children's visits at jails and development of interventions that prepare children and other family members for visits. In the present report we focus on the observational data collected from children visiting in the jail setting and their implications for policy and practice.

Based on our observations, there appear to be both positive and negative components to young children's experiences of video and barrier visits in jail settings. Because video visits were conducted in a nonsecure part of each corrections facility, fewer security procedures were required for video visits, and there were shorter wait times for families using the video visits compared to barrier visits. However, the length of video visits was shorter, and video visits often ended abruptly with the screen turning off without any warning to children. Although barrier visits were associated with longer wait times and more intense security procedures, visits lasted longer, providing children and their caregivers with more time for conversation. Yet the longer that children were in the corrections facility, the more clingy and distressed they became, possibly reflecting increased stress levels. Although children's behaviors (i.e., behavioral dysregulation, activity level, and emotional lability) did not differ across type of visit, children exhibited more dysregulation in the jail setting compared to the home. Jail settings, especially experiencing security procedures and long wait times, can be stressful and fatigue-inducing for some young children. However, few children expressed overt fear or distress during the observation period. Most children alternated between expressing serious and happy affect (e.g., smiling or laughing).

Although visiting a parent incarcerated in jail can be related to increases in dysregulated child behavior, visits also are a chance for children to express positive emotions and love to incarcerated parents. All children expressed happiness when seeing their incarcerated parents and most of them expressed loving sentiments to their parents. Caregiver support during the visit appeared vital, as children stayed in close proximity to their caregivers and engaged in an increasing level of contact maintenance toward their caregivers the longer the visit lasted, suggesting a heighted activation of the child's attachment system as the visit unfolded. Activation of a child's attachment system is often caused by stress (Ainsworth, Blehar, Waters, & Wall, 1978; Bowlby, 1982) and gold standard assessments of attachment in infants and toddlers rely on inducing mild stress. We conclude that behaviors that we observed in the jail setting were mildly stressful for children, on average, and required support from loving adults.

Activation of a child's attachment system within the jail visitation setting has implications for caregivers, who may already be stressed by the visit as well as factors (e.g., financial situation, caring for child, custody issues, having a family member in jail, other stressors). Caregivers may or may not know how to respond to children's bids for attention or their increased clinginess during the visit, or they may not be able to focus intently on the child's needs, especially if they are visiting the jailed individual based on their own reasons and needs. Despite these factors, caregivers sometimes prompted young children about what to say to the incarcerated parent, thus facilitating the content of the visit and the relationship between the incarcerated parent and the child. One unexpected observation related to how often children were exposed to the visits of people sitting next to them during both video and Plexiglas visits, which may present an unexpected lack of privacy for children, caregivers and incarcerated parents. Many caregivers were unsure of how to handle such situations, whereas others appeared unaware of their child's attentional focus during segments of the visit.

At the three jails that collaborated on the study, corrections staff regularly commented on how the visits seemed chaotic when young children were present. Staff remarked that during the waiting period and visits, young children often ran around or rolled around on the floor, and many staff members indicated that they would like to see the visits occur in a calmer, more orderly manner. Personnel in corrections facilities are more likely to meet such goals when they begin to understand how children and families experience visits with incarcerated individuals. Thus, the present study provides an initial contribution to our understanding of young children's experiences of visitation.

As in any study, there are numerous limitations, and the current findings need replication and extension to prison settings and other jail settings to be viewed as robust.

The present study's generalizability was limited by the small sample size and focus on jails in only one state. It is unknown if there were unobserved jail characteristics that led them to opt for one type of visit over another (e.g., age of jail). Moreover, ratings of children's behavior occurred live in the jail setting, so researchers were not blind to the type of jail visit (e.g., video or Plexiglas), and training and establishing inter-rater reliability was slightly more challenging than when videos are used in observational research. In the future, time sampling could be used to determine how long children stayed in a particular state, rather than use of more global rating or presence/absence of behaviors. Because of the use of in vivo ratings, researchers focused on the behavior of children rather than the behavior of caregivers or incarcerated parents. In the future, it would be beneficial to rate how caregivers and incarcerated parents respond to children and help shape the visit experience for children. Additional data are needed to complement the focus on observations in the jail setting. In the present study, we also interviewed jailed parents and caregivers and collected much child-focused data in the home environment. This information will be forthcoming in future publications as we complete data collection for this project.

Despite the limitations, these findings have implications for intervention and policy. We briefly mention several such implications here, although Poehlmann-Tynan (2015) goes into more depth about them in the Summary and Recommendations chapter of this monograph, including discussion of the materials that Sesame Workshop (2013) developed for children with incarcerated parents. The most obvious recommendation that we see coming from these data is the need for child-friendly visitation in corrections facilities. Child-friendly visits (Dallaire, Poehlmann, & Loper, 2011) can be defined as providing positive, safe, friendly environments for visits, fostering open communication among caregivers, children, incarcerated parents, and supportive professionals, adequately preparing children for visits, facilitating parent–child contact between visits, and supporting incarcerated parents during the process. Often, children who visit at corrections facilities appear happy to see their parents and want to engage with them. Yet the physical and social context of incarceration often does not allow for a parent–child connection that is without some stressors. Preparing children for visits and helping caregivers understand how to support children effectively during the process are important, even when security procedures or non-contact visits are unavoidable. Another recommendation is for jails to collect data about the parental status of inmates during the intake or assessment process so that together we can determine how many children are affected, how old they are, if the jailed parent is still involved in their children's lives, and if the child is likely to visit. With such data, we can develop a better picture of the parenting needs of jailed individuals as well as the presence of vulnerable children in various communities. The process of identification is often a critical first step in developing needs assessments and more resources for vulnerable families.

Additional recommendations relate to supporting caregivers, who are responsible for the care and well-being of children during parental incarceration. In our previous studies, we have found that caregiver poverty and mental health (e.g., depressive symptoms) is related to the quality of the home environment that they provide to children as well as children's attachment to the caregiver and cognitive development. Caregivers often take responsibility for talking to children about the parent's incarceration, sometimes deciding whether or not to tell children the truth or to make up a "cover" story or say nothing. Caregivers regulate visits between children and their incarcerated parents and are often the individuals who are there to support the children during the visitation process at the jail or prison. For young children, caregivers are frequently the adult who places or accepts phone calls to or from the incarcerated parent and they also get and read the mail to children or send children's notes, pictures, and drawings to the incarcerated parent. The importance of caregivers in children's lives during parental incarceration cannot be overstated. And even more importantly, these caregivers often need assistance because of the many stressors and risks that they face. Although there is a growing recognition about problems related to mass incarceration and its collateral consequences for families, there is more that society can do to support affected children and their caregivers.

Future research on this topic should examine the potential stress process that may occur in some children during contact and non-contact visits with incarcerated parents using physiological as well as behavioral measures with children, caregivers, and parents. Inclusion of research focusing on parent–child interaction across multiple settings when parents are incarcerated is important because it is a key proximal process. Proximal processes have a potent effect on young children, as they reflect the child's common, lived experiences. Future research should also examine the reunification process between children and their jailed parents following release from prison or jail, as family interactions may be important for children's adjustment during this transition (Baker, McHale, Strozier, & Cecil, 2010).

Acknowledgements This research was supported by grants from the National Institutes of Health (R21HD068581, PI: Poehlmann and P30HD03352, PI: Mailick) and the University of Wisconsin. The content is solely the responsibility of the authors and does not necessarily represent the official views of the NIH. Special thanks to Racine, Dane, and Sauk County Sheriff's offices and jail staff for their support of the project; to Beverlee Baker, Susan Bulla, and Sue Nagelkerk from University of Wisconsin-Extension for their work on the project; to numerous undergraduate students for assistance with data collection and coding; and to the families who participated in this research.

3.5 Appendix A

Jail-Prison Observation Checklist

General Information

Site: _____ CG w/targeted child: _____ # of other children & age(s): _____

Visit occurs through: ☐ Closed circuit TV ☐ Plexiglas ☐ Face-to-Face

Number of Adults in Waiting Area: _____ Number of Adults in Visit Area: _____
Number of Children in Waiting Area: _____ Number of Children in Visit Area: _____

Time Checked-In: _____ Time Called for Visit: _____ Time Visit Ended: _____
                                  Total Wait Time: _____ Total Visit Time: _____

Interaction with staff: *rate on a 1 to 5 scale, check box on right*	Security	Wait	Visit
1 = Negative (minimal communication, negative affect, confrontation)	☐	☐	☐
2 = Moderately negative (terse interaction)	☐	☐	☐
3 = Neutral	☐	☐	☐
4 = Moderately positive (slightly friendly)	☐	☐	☐
5 = Positive (e.g., clear communication, positive affect)	☐	☐	☐

Child affect: *check any that occur; circle predominant one*	Security	Wait	Visit
Tired (rubbing eyes, yawn, sleepy, sleeping, put head down, faking, slouched posture)	☐	☐	☐
Confused or somber (furrowed brow, visual scanning, serious look on face)	☐	☐	☐
Fearful (raised brow, wide eyes, pursed mouth, shaking/shivering, hiding hands using clothes)	☐	☐	☐
Sad (turned down mouth with neutral brow, crying, defeated posture)	☐	☐	☐
Happy or excited (smiling, laughing, jumping, dancing)	☐	☐	☐
Angry (furrowed brow with turned down mouth, scowl, yelling, aggressive language, defiant)	☐	☐	☐
Serious/somber (stoic, expressionless, lack of language, distracted)	☐	☐	☐
Self-soothing behaviors (sucking thumb or object, twirling hair, rocking)	☐	☐	☐
Anxious (fidgety, apprehensive, pacing, worried, uneasy)	☐	☐	☐

Child attachment behaviors toward caregiver: *check any that occur*	Security	Wait	Visit
Staying in close proximity to adult	☐	☐	☐
Holding adult's hand	☐	☐	☐
Clinging to or other physical contact with adult (other than holding hand, hugging)	☐	☐	☐
Crying (holding back tears)	☐	☐	☐
Whining	☐	☐	☐
Pushing adult away	☐	☐	☐
Avoiding adult (sitting elsewhere)	☐	☐	☐
Hitting adult (swings at adult, shove)	☐	☐	☐

SECURITY PROCEDURES

Safety procedures: *check any that occur*   Yes   No
- Metal detector?   ☐   ☐
- Frisking or patting down adults?   ☐   ☐
- Frisking or patting down children?   ☐   ☐
- Remove shoes, belts, other pieces of clothing?   ☐   ☐
- Search of purses, diapers?   ☐   ☐
- Asking to see parent's ID, child's birth certificate?   ☐   ☐

VISIT WITH INCARCERATED PARENT

Child behaviors toward incarcerated parent: *check any that occur*   Yes   No
- Paying visual attention to incarcerated parent?   ☐   ☐
- Verbalizing to incarcerated parent?   ☐   ☐
- Listening to what incarcerated parent says?   ☐   ☐
- Responding to what incarcerated parent says nonverbally?   ☐   ☐
- Avoiding incarcerated parent?   ☐   ☐
- Looking at other visitors or other incarcerated parents/monitors?   ☐   ☐

Child emotions toward incarcerated parent: *check any that occur*   Yes   No
- Fearful   ☐   ☐
- Sad   ☐   ☐
- Happy   ☐   ☐
- Excited   ☐   ☐
- Somber   ☐   ☐
- Angry   ☐   ☐
- Loving   ☐   ☐
- Confused   ☐   ☐
- Crying   ☐   ☐
- Whining   ☐   ☐

GLOBAL FACILITY RATINGS

Noise level: *rate on a 1 to 5 scale, check box on right*
- 1 = Quiet ☐
- 2 = Mostly quiet ☐
- 3 = Modest (murmuring voices, can hear person next to you speaking in normal voice) ☐
- 4 = Moderately loud (modest, with some instances of loud noise) ☐
- 5 = Loud (difficult to hear the person next to you when they speak in a normal voice) ☐

Cleanliness: *rate on a 1 to 5 scale with circle*
- 1 = Very clean ☐
- 2 = Moderately clean ☐
- 3 = Somewhat clean and somewhat dirty ☐
- 4 = Moderately dirty ☐
- 5 = Very dirty ☐

3 Young Children's Behavioral and Emotional Reactions to Plexiglas and Video... 57

Are there materials available for children to play with?   Yes ☐   No ☐

If so, note what and where: _____

GLOBAL CHILD RATINGS

<u>Child's overall activity level</u>: *rate on a 1 to 5 scale, check box on right*

1 = very low activity; stays in one place most of the time or moves slowly ☐

2 = low activity level ☐

3 = modest activity level; appears to have normal amount and speed of activity for age ☐

4 = high activity level ☐

5 = very high activity level; moves around most of the time; moves quickly (run, climb) ☐

<u>Child's overall level of behavioral dysregulation</u>: *rate on a 1 to 5 scale, check box on right*

1 = very high behavioral regulation; seems very tightly in control of own behaviors and has no problems containing self in situation, does not need reminders to behave ☐

2 = high behavioral regulation; in control of own behaviors much of time; lapses are minor ☐

3 = modest level of dysregulation for age (what one would expect); may have moments with some dysregulation but quickly recovers with age-appropriate adult intervention ☐

4 = high level of dysregulation; appears out of control some times; recovering takes time ☐

5 = very high level of behavioral dysregulation; appeared out of control or emotionally or behaviorally "all over the place" most of the time; seemed to have difficulty containing self in situation; recovery is fleeting or takes a long time to achieve ☐

<u>Child's overall level of emotional lability</u>: *rate on a 1 to 5 scale, check box on right*

1 = very low emotional lability; very limited or restricted range of emotions (only one main emotion observed during the whole visit) ☐

2 = low emotional lability; shows more than one primary emotion but slow transition between emotions; some restriction of range ☐

3 = expresses modest range of emotions for age; does not quickly change from one emotion to another ☐

4 = high emotional lability; wide range of emotions or intensity ☐

5 = very high emotional lability; very wide range of intense emotions expressed; quickly changes from one emotion to another ☐

CAREGIVER IMPRESSIONS

Ask caregiver: Was this visit similar to, or different from, other visits the child has had with his/her incarcerated parent?

OBSERVER's NOTES:

References

Ainsworth, M. D. S., Blehar, M., Waters, E., & Wall, S. (1978). *Patterns of attachment: A psychological study of the strange situation*. Hillsdale, NJ: Erlbaum.

Arditti, J. A. (2012). *Parental incarceration and the family: Psychological and social effects of imprisonment on children, parents, and caregivers*. New York: NYU Press.

Arditti, J. A., Lambert-Shute, J., & Joest, K. (2003). Saturday morning at the jail: Implications of incarceration for families and children. *Family Relations, 52*(3), 195–204. doi:10.1111/j.1741-3729.2003.00195.x.

Baker, J., McHale, J., Strozier, A., & Cecil, D. (2010). Mother–grandmother coparenting relationships in families with incarcerated mothers: A pilot investigation. *Family Process, 49*(2), 165–184.

Bowlby, J. (1982). *Attachment: Volume 1: Attachment* (2nd ed.). New York: Basic Books.

Center for Disease Control. (2009). Adverse childhood experiences reported by adults—five states. *Morbidity and Mortality Weekly Report, 59*(49), 1609–1613.

Dallaire, D. H., Ciccone, A., & Wilson, L. C. (2012). The family drawings of at-risk children: Concurrent relations with contact with incarcerated parents, caregiver behavior, and stress. *Attachment & Human Development, 14*(2), 161–183.

Dallaire, D., Poehlmann, J., & Loper, A. (2011). Issues and recommendations related to children's visitation and contact with incarcerated parents. United Nations Committee on the Rights of the Child, Day of General Discussion, Children of Incarcerated Parents. http://www2.ohchr.org/english/bodies/crc/discussion2011_submissions.htm

Eddy, J. M., & Poehlmann, J. (2010). *Children of incarcerated parents: A handbook for researchers and practitioners*. Washington, D C: Urban Institute Press.

Glaze, L. E., & Maruschak, L. M. (2008). *Parents in prison and their minor children*. Washington, DC: U.S. Department of Justice, Office of Justice Programs.

Kemper, K. J., & Rivara, F. P. (1993). Parents in jail. *Pediatrics, 92*, 261–264.

Minton, T. D., & Golinelli, D. (2014). *Jail inmates at midyear 2013: Statistical tables. Bureau of Justice Statistics*. Washington, DC: U.S. Department of Justice.

Murray, J., & Farrington, D. P. (2008). Parental imprisonment: Long-lasting effects on boys' internalizing problems through the life course. *Development and Psychopathology, 20*(1), 273–290. doi:10.1017/S0954579408000138.

Murray, J., Farrington, D. P., Sekol, I., & Olsen, R. F. (2009). Effects of parental imprisonment on child antisocial behaviour and mental health: A systematic review. *Campbell Systematic Reviews, 4*, 1–105. Oslo, Norway: Campbell Collaboration. doi:10.4073/csr.2009.4.

Osborne Association. (2012). *New York initiative for children of incarcerated parents fact sheet*. Brooklyn: The Osborne Association.

Poehlmann, J. (2012). Jail-prison observation checklist. See Appendix A. University of Wisconsin-Madison.

Poehlmann, J., Dallaire, D. H., Loper, A. B., & Shear, L. D. (2010). Children's contact with their incarcerated parents: Research findings and recommendations. *American Psychologist, 65*(6), 575–598. doi:10.1037/a0020279.

Poehlmann, J., & Eddy, J. M. (Eds.) (2013). Relationship processes and resilience in children with incarcerated parents. *Monographs of the Society for Research in Child Development, 78*(3): 75–93.

San Francisco Children of Incarcerated Parents Partnership. (2005). Children of incarcerated parents: A bill of rights. Retrieved from www.sfcipp.org

Sesame Workshop and Advisors: Adalist-Estrin, A., Burton, C. F., Gaynes, E., Harris, K. E., & Poehlmann, J. (2013). Little children, big challenges: Incarceration. Retrieved from http://www.sesamestreet.org/parents/topicsandactivities/toolkits/incarceration

Chapter 4
Associations Among Mother–Child Contact, Parenting Stress, and Mother and Child Adjustment Related to Incarceration

Heather H. McClure, Joann Wu Shortt, J. Mark Eddy, Alice Holmes, Stan Van Uum, Evan Russell, Gideon Koren, Lisa Sheeber, Betsy Davis, J. Josh Snodgrass, and Charles R. Martinez Jr.

4.1 Introduction

The number of incarcerated women has increased dramatically in recent years, doubling between 1991 and 2008 (Glaze & Maruschak, 2008; West & Sabol, 2008). The majority of women in prison are mothers of dependent children. The percentages are highest for women aged 25–34 years, with about 80 % in state prison and 75 % in federal prison having children under the age of 18 years. Advocates have

---

H.H. McClure
Center for Equity Promotion, University of Oregon, Eugene, OR, USA

J.W. Shortt (✉) • A. Holmes
Oregon Social Learning Center, 10 Shelton McMurphy Blvd., Eugene, OR 97401, USA
e-mail: joanns@oslc.org

J.M. Eddy, Ph.D.
Partners for Our Children, School of Social Work, University of Washington,
UW Tower, UW Mailbox 359476, Seattle, WA 98195-9476, USA
e-mail: jmarke@uw.edu

S. Van Uum • E. Russell
Department of Medicine, Western University, London, ON, Canada

G. Koren
The Ivey Chair in Molecular Toxicology, Western University, London, ON, Canada

L. Sheeber • B. Davis
Oregon Research Institute, Eugene, OR, USA

J.J. Snodgrass
Department of Anthropology, University of Oregon, Eugene, OR, USA

C.R. Martinez Jr.
Center for Equity Promotion, University of Oregon, Eugene, OR, USA
Department of Educational Methodology, Policy and Leadership, University of Oregon, Eugene, OR, USA

© Springer International Publishing Switzerland 2015
J. Poehlmann-Tynan (ed.), *Children's Contact with Incarcerated Parents*,
SpringerBriefs in Psychology, DOI 10.1007/978-3-319-16625-4_4

estimated that up to ten million children (1 in 8 children in the U.S.) have experienced parental incarceration at some point in their lives (San Francisco Partnership for Incarcerated Parents, 2003a). A growing body of literature suggests that the children of incarcerated parents are more emotionally and behaviorally vulnerable than their peers (Eddy & Poehlmann, 2010; Poehlmann & Eddy, 2013). In a recent meta-analysis, experiencing parental incarceration was related to children's increased risk for the display of antisocial behavior in particular (Murray, Farrington, & Sekol, 2012).

For the children of incarcerated mothers, there are many possible reasons for increased vulnerability and risk. Prior to incarceration, mothers may have faced substantial challenges to creating home environments that are optimal for their children's development. These challenges are often rooted in a lifetime of disadvantage and related stress exposure, including growing up in poverty and in a single-parent household, dropping out of school, experiencing physical or sexual abuse, having at least one immediate family member who was incarcerated, having a parent who abused alcohol or drugs, and becoming a parent at an early age relative to other women (Greenfield & Snell, 2000). As adults, substance use dependence, posttraumatic stress, and depression—all conditions with a higher lifetime prevalence among incarcerated than non-incarcerated women (Travis & Waul, 2003)—can further challenge effective parenting and increase risk for their children's development of problem behaviors particularly when compounded by present-day poverty, residential instability, and limited vocational training and work opportunities (Kjellstrand, Cearley, Eddy, Foney, & Martinez, 2012; Kjellstrand & Eddy, 2011a, 2011b). Given this potential pile-up of adversity, incarceration can be construed as a continuation or exacerbation of stressful life experiences for mothers and for their children and families.

In addition to the risks posed by pre-existing adversity in many families, maternal incarceration often means the addition of at least one other risk, a disruption in caretaking. The transitional period following release may be challenging for both mother and child due to minimal contact and related disruptions in the relationship (Poehlmann, 2005) and mothers' experiences of prisonization that can challenge mothers' resumption of their parenting role. In a national study, over 64 % of children of incarcerated parents lived with their mother before arrest or just prior to incarceration, and 52 % had a mother who was the primary financial supporter for the family (Glaze & Maruschak, 2008). While mothers are incarcerated, most children (over 75 % in the same study) live with a non-parental relative or friend, usually a grandparent. Only 37 % live with the other parent, and a significant portion of those children also live with another caretaker as well. Given that many children lived with their mothers before prison, it is not surprising that the vast majority of mothers (85 %) had some contact with their children while incarcerated with over half (56 %) having contact at least weekly.

Contact between imprisoned adults, their children, and other family members has long been an area of interest to researchers, practitioners, and corrections administrators. Most notably, an oft cited study of prison administrative records found that frequent visits did not improve the behavior of men while incarcerated, but were related to better parole plans, better chances of being paroled, and doing better after release while on parole (Holt & Miller, 1972). For inmates with no visitors and no correspondence, 12 % had "serious" difficulties during their first year on parole versus only 2 % who had three or more visitors. Further, while 50 % of inmates with no visitors had no parole difficulties, approximately 70 % of those with three or more visitors had no difficulties. Holt and Miller put special emphasis in their conclusions on the value of family visits during prison. More recent studies using much larger samples and including both men and women inmates have found similar positive associations between the number of visits inmates have, including those with various family members, and post-release outcomes such as recidivism (e.g., Bales & Mears, 2008; Minnesota Department of Corrections, 2011). Whether these findings are related to contact or are due to pre-existing differences prior to incarceration is unclear.

As many mothers are caregivers to their children both prior to and following incarceration (Hagan & Coleman, 2001), the impact of mother-child contact is of particular interest. Such contact may occur through visits, phone calls, or letters. Poehlmann, Dallaire, Loper, and Shear (2010) identified 36 studies conducted after 1998 on incarcerated parent–child contact; of these, nine studies reported on incarcerated maternal outcomes (seven studies found positive and two studies found negative maternal effects) and nine studies reported on child outcomes (four studies found positive, two studies found negative, and three studies found both positive and negative effects). The most common positive outcome examined for incarcerated mothers was improved parent adjustment, such as less maternal "distress," fewer depressive symptoms, more empathy, and less parenting "stress". No negative impacts of contact on these types of parent adjustment were reported. Positive outcomes for children associated with more contact included more secure attachment (among infants), less child depression and somatic complaints, fewer child school drop outs and suspensions, and fewer feelings of alienation from the incarcerated parent. Negative outcomes for children associated with more contact included insecure attachment and behavioral problems. Interestingly, only two studies examined the impact of mother-child contact on recidivism: one found positive effects (Carlson, 1998) and the other negative effects (Bales & Mears, 2008).

The focus on parental stress in the literature on inmate family contact builds on the broader literature on the impact of imprisonment on the mental health of prisoners and the direct consequences of such on their family members (Travis & Waul, 2003). This work points to the ways in which requisite coping strategies developed in response to stressors that are specific to prisons and prison culture can result in hypervigilance, interpersonal distrust and suspicion, emotional overcontrol, alienation, psychological distancing, social withdrawal and isolation, the incorporation of exploitative norms of prisoner culture, and a diminished sense of self-worth and personal value (Haney, 2003). Inmates with prior histories of trauma may be particularly vulnerable to posttraumatic stress reactions to imprisonment (Herman, 1992; Masten & Garmezy, 1985).

Exposure to prison life may significantly transform the individual. This is especially true of individuals who enter prison at an early age (Haney, 2003).

Coping responses learned while in prison may interfere with an incarcerated mother's transition to her home, impede her successful reintegration into community and work settings, and challenge her ability to resume her role with family and children. Former inmates' experiences of the unique set of psychological adaptations that typically occur in response to the extraordinary demands of prison life (Peat & Winfree, 1992) may not only alter habits of thinking, feeling, and acting, but may also influence their physiology and stress responsivity (Sapolsky, 2004), with unknown consequences for that individual's reintegration experience into the community.

In recent years, investigations of stress, or the psychological and physical reactions of individuals to environmental stressors, have been undertaken to better understand the links between exposure to specific conditions and various individual and family outcomes (Gibbons, Gerrard, Cleveland, Wills, & Brody, 2004). Many researchers are also examining stress-related coping, as exposure to stressors have been shown to influence health by directly causing physiological changes, and indirectly by increasing the likelihood of risky and unhealthy coping behaviors such as drug use (Gibbons et al., 2010). Recent studies have illuminated pathways between persistent exposure to stressors and physiological responses, such as dysregulated cortisol production, that can prime the body to be more physically reactive in potentially stressful social situations, thus reducing the capacity of an individual to remain attentive, think clearly, and learn (Gunnar & Donzella, 2002; Gunnar & Vazquez, 2001). Heightened stress reactivity can create vulnerability for poor adjustment, including depression and anxiety, social and emotional problems, and learning difficulties. These challenges can be compounded for parents and children when parents engage in unhealthy coping behaviors, including smoking, alcohol, and drug use and abuse, overeating, social isolation, and reduced help-seeking (Gibbons et al., 2010; Williams & Mohammed, 2009). Hence, stressors can challenge parent adjustment, diminish effective parenting practices, and thereby threaten healthy child adjustment.

Despite the potential relations between stress and the adjustment of incarcerated parents and their children, few studies involving incarcerated populations have conducted in depth examinations of inmate stress. Notably, all of the studies included in the Poehlmann et al. (2010) review included self-report measures of stress. As an initial step towards broadening the knowledge base on stress and incarcerated mothers, in the study reported here, we integrated the neurophysiological stress marker cortisol into a battery of self-report measures of maternal psychosocial functioning. In doing so, our hope was to gain deeper insights into the relations among maternal stress and mental health and children's adjustment.

Cortisol is the primary glucocorticoid hormone in humans, and the product of activity of the hypothalamic-pituitary-adrenal (HPA) axis that regulates the body's stress response, mobilizing energy stores and modulating the functioning of the immune system (Hellhammer, Wüst, & Kudielka, 2009; Sapolsky, Romero, & Munck, 2000). Cortisol typically has a strong diurnal rhythm, with highest levels in the early morning and lowest levels in the late evening. Over time, everyday negative experiences can contribute to atypical cortisol fluctuation with either high or blunted cortisol levels in the morning and flatter diurnal curves over the day; downstream effects can include the development and/or progression of major depression, obesity, Type 2 diabetes, and cardiovascular disease (McEwen & Wingfield, 2003; Rosmond, 2001). Though cortisol is most commonly assayed using saliva or urine, we were unable to collect these types of samples and transport them out of the prison setting, but we were allowed to collect samples of hair. Hair analysis has been used for decades to monitor exposure to drugs and other exogenous compounds. In recent years, researchers have grown increasingly interested in quantifying endogenously produced compounds through hair (Russell, Koren, Rieder, & Van Uum, 2012). According to Russell et al. (2012) of research involving cortisol in hair, findings from clinical and community studies support its reliability as an objective biomarker of stress, including psychosocial stress. Higher hair cortisol concentrations have been reported in pregnant women with higher scores on the Perceived Stress Scale (Kalra, Einarson, Karskov, Van Uum, & Koren, 2007), patients with chronic pain compared with patients without pain (Van Uum et al., 2008), individuals who are unemployed compared with employed subjects (Dettenborn, Tietze, Bruckner, & Kirschbaum, 2010), neonates in intensive care compared with babies born at term (Yamada et al., 2007), and in individuals three months prior to being diagnosed with acute myocardial infarction (Pereg et al., 2010). The relationship between hair cortisol and high stress exposure is not always a positive one, however. For example, patients with generalized anxiety disorder have been shown to have higher perceived stress scores and lower cortisol than controls, providing evidence of hypocortisolemia, or the downregulation of the HPA axis (Steudte et al., 2011), a physiological attempt to calm an overactive system and maintain homeostasis. As posttraumatic stress disorder is more common among incarcerated women, findings such as these indicate that study participants' lifetime exposure to stressors might translate into cortisol values that are either substantially lower or higher than those of other community samples.

4.1.1 Research Questions

In the present report, we examine associations between mother-child contact, self-report and biological measures of maternal stress and adjustment, and caregiver report of child adjustment during and after maternal imprisonment. Past work in the area of incarceration related to parent and child functioning has been hampered by limited measurement strategies and lack of replication. Here, we examine three sets of research questions:

1. How do average levels of mothers' cortisol change over time, both while in prison and after release from prison? Do average levels of parenting stress and maternal adjustment (i.e., emotion dysregulation and depressive and other mental health symptoms) change in similar ways to mothers' cortisol across time?

2. What are the relations among mothers' cortisol, parenting stress, and maternal adjustment, and between maternal adjustment and children's adjustment (i.e., emotion regulation ability, internalizing and externalizing symptoms, and social skills)?
3. What are the relations between mother-child contact during and after a prison sentence and (a) mothers' cortisol, parenting stress, adjustment, and recidivism, and (b) children's adjustment?

4.2 Methods

4.2.1 Study Overview

The current investigation was conducted as an exploratory study within a larger intervention development study (*Emotions*: *Taking care of yourself when you and your child return home* [*Project Home*]; Shortt, Eddy, Sheeber, & Davis, 2014). Funded by the National Institutes of Health, Project Home was designed to provide incarcerated mothers with tools to effectively regulate their own emotions and to parent in ways that encourage their children's effective emotion regulation. By strengthening parenting and emotional skills through participation in the *Emotions Program*, Project Home aimed to help incarcerated parents and families to reduce stress associated with incarceration and transition from prison. The project extended work begun in a randomized controlled trial of the *Parenting Inside Out* parent management training program for incarcerated mothers and fathers (Eddy, Martinez, & Burraston, 2013). Project Home involved 47 mothers (at baseline) incarcerated at the only women's state correctional facility in Oregon, with assignment of participants to either an intervention (i.e., the *Emotions Program*) or control condition. Mothers in both conditions were assessed at baseline, prior to the *Emotions Program* (T1); after the *Emotions Program*, while still in prison (T2); and at 6 months, after release back to the community (T3) (Shortt et al., 2014). Primary caregivers were assessed regarding children's adjustment at T1 and T3. The study was approved by the Oregon Social Learning Center's (OSLC) Institutional Review Board (IRB), the Oregon Department of Corrections Research Committee, and the U.S. Department of Health and Human Services, Office for Human Research Protections. The OSLC IRB monitored the progress of the study.

4.2.2 Participants

As has been reported elsewhere (Shortt et al., 2014), participants were 47 mothers aged 32.8 years old on average ($SD=6.9$). Thirty of the children's caregivers also participated in the study. One-third of mothers (32 %) identified as racial or ethnic minority (more than one race 15 %, Latina 11 %, American Indian 4 %, and African American 2 %). Mothers' average prison sentence was 3.6 years (range 1–9 years), and crimes included assault, burglary, delivery of methamphetamine, and manslaughter, among others. While mothers were incarcerated, their children lived with caregivers an average of 108 miles from the prison (range 11–972 miles). The children ($n=30$) were on average 7.3 years old ($SD=2.7$) and the majority were boys (62 %). Forty-two percent of children were identified as ethnic or racial minorities. Nearly all women (96 %) were the biological mothers of their children, most had lived with their children before incarceration (74 %, full or part time), and a majority had had contact with their children in the month before the study began (53 %). The majority of mothers (87 %) were single or never married, separated or divorced, or widowed before incarceration; did not complete high school (60 %); were unemployed (51 %); had been arrested five or more times as adults (63 %); and had juvenile detainment records (53 %). After release from prison, less than half (42 %) of mothers returned to live with their children (full or part time), though most (82 %) were in contact with their children in the past month. During the 6 month period of post-prison observation, 68 % of mothers were unemployed, and 21 % were detained at some point.

4.2.3 Recruitment and Retention

Prerequisites for participation included being within 6 months of release from prison and the prior completion of the group-based *Parenting Inside Out* parent management training program (2013, Eddy et al., 2008; Schiffmann, Eddy, Martinez, Leve, & Newton, 2008). If individuals were convicted of crimes against children or any type of sex offense, they were not eligible for *Parenting Inside Out*, and hence were not eligible for this study. Participating mothers were recruited using standard procedures that are used in the prison system to inform inmates about intervention programs, educational classes, and research projects (e.g., through prison newspapers, announcements in public gatherings, bulletin-board postings). Once a mother signaled her potential interest in participation, project staff met with her to provide an overview of the project and to answer any questions. Informed consent was obtained at this time. Mothers who consented to participate in the project also signed a release form giving study staff permission to contact their child's caregiver. Of eligible mothers, 87 % were recruited to participate; the recruitment rate of caregivers was 64 %. As for participant retention over the study, at T2, 100 % of mothers completed an assessment. By T3, 6 months after release, the retention rate was 81 % for mothers and 83 % for caregivers.

4.2.4 Procedures

Project Home involved a quasi-experimental design in which mothers were assigned to either the *Emotions Program* group ($n=29$) or to the comparison group ($n=18$), whose members did not receive additional parenting services beyond the Parenting Inside Out training that occurred prior to this study. Three waves of assessment were conducted with mothers including at baseline prior to the *Emotions Program* (T1), after the *Emotions Program* while mothers were still in prison before release (T2), and 6 months after release back to the community (T3). Caregiver reports on the children were obtained at T1 and T3. Assessments for mothers comprised administering a battery of questions (see Section 4.2.5) via an in-person interview as well as collecting a hair sample and measuring participants' height, weight, waist circumference, and blood pressure. In prison, the interview and hair sample collection were conducted in a private room. Out of prison, interviews were conducted in a private setting, most commonly in the homes of participants. Mothers were compensated $25 for completing the T1 assessment in prison, $25 for completing the T2 assessment in prison before release, and $50 for completing the T3 assessment after release. No additional compensation was provided to participants involved in the intervention. Interviews with caregivers also were conducted in a private setting, most often the caregivers' homes. Caregivers were compensated $50 at T1 and $50 at T3 for completing reports on the children.

Hair sample collection and cortisol analysis. Hair samples were collected from participants following the protocol designed by Van Uum and colleagues (see Russell et al., 2012). According to this protocol, a sample of hair was cut as close to the scalp as possible at the base of the vertex posterior of the head. As the preservation of cortisol in hair does not require special storage prior to analysis, each hair sample was affixed to sample paper and stored in an envelope in a secure area only accessible to project staff until it was mailed to the Van Uum lab. According to Russell et al., 2012, hair grows an average of 1 cm per month with the most proximal 1 cm segment to the scalp reflecting the last month's cortisol patterns. The analysis of cortisol in hair requires 10–15 mg of hair per section being measured, and hair cortisol analysis was performed according to procedures described elsewhere (Russell et al., 2012). We obtained 40 hair samples at T1, 36 samples at T2[1], and 25 samples at T3; two T3 samples were not analyzed because they did not contain enough hair.

Additional considerations regarding the collection and analysis of hair samples from incarcerated women. It took several months for the Oregon Department of Corrections to approve the study's request to collect biological measures. This permission, however, did not allow study assessors to bring scissors into the facility. Instead, assessors checked out prison scissors at each visit; these small child size craft scissors had short, rounded, and dull blades, and were used for art and craft projects. Though serviceable, these scissors were not ideal for the delicate and quick collection of hair close to the scalp. The collection of hair is among the least invasive ways to collect biological material for the analysis of cortisol (Russell et al., 2012). Nevertheless, hair took on special significance for many women in prison with implications for hair collection procedures.

---

[1] Unique to the analysis of cortisol in hair, specific sections of the same hair sample can be assayed to obtain cortisol levels during different periods of time. In this manner, T2 cortisol levels were obtained for a few participants that did not provide a hair sample at T2 using their hair sample provided at T3.

At T1, 81 % of participants initially signed informed consent forms agreeing to our collection of a hair sample. When the assessor began to collect hair from the first two participants, however, their clear discomfort with the process led to the addition of several steps involving the clear description of each next step in the procedure and ongoing requests for permission to proceed. Among reasons participants provided for their refusal included fear that we would analyze DNA (despite assessor assurances that we would not), being Native American for whom hair is sacred, and concern about having a bald spot that would not grow in, or that would grow just enough by the time of reunification with family members to appear "spiky." Several women requested that the sample to be cut be made smaller; assessors responded to these requests while also attempting to collect a quantity that still met minimum requirements for analysis (10–15 mg of hair 1 cm in length). Upon reflection, it became clear that, for many incarcerated women, their hair was one of the few personal possessions they were allowed to keep, rendering many women highly protective of and strongly identified with their hair. This appeared especially true for women who had served sentences of many years. Some of the mothers had not cut their hair in several years and their hair was extremely long. Despite the small diameter of the sample (thickness of a dime or 1.35 mm), for women with long hair the length of the hair made the slender sample look like a large quantity.

4.2.5 *Psychosocial Measures*

The interview focused on key constructs including mothers' parenting stress and adjustment, including emotion dysregulation and mental health, as well as demographics. Mothers also were asked about contact with their child, including whether they lived with their child prior to incarceration and after release, and the type(s) and frequency of contact with their child while in prison and after release. Mothers also were asked questions regarding events related to criminal behavior, such as how long they had been incarcerated and whether they had been detained post-release. Caregivers were asked about children's adjustment such as their abilities to regulate emotions, internalizing and externalizing symptoms, and social skills. The interview included questions from several standardized questionnaires that have been used in prior studies.

Mothers' parenting stress. Mothers' parenting stress (reverse of parenting satisfaction and efficacy) was measured via the 10-item *Being a Parent* scale, which was originally adapted for the FastTrack project (McMahon & Lengua, 1996; example item "Being a parent makes you tense and anxious"). High scores indicated high levels of parenting stress. Across T1 to T3, Cronbach alphas varied from 0.77 to 0.78.

Mothers' adjustment. Maternal emotion dysregulation was measured using the 36-item *Difficulties in Emotion Regulation Scale* (Gratz & Roemer, 2004; example item: "When I'm upset, it takes me a long time to feel better"). Across T1 to T3, the Cronbach alphas ranged from 0.94 to 0.95. Mothers' depressive symptoms were assessed using the 20-item *Center for Epidemiologic Studies Depression Scale* (Radloff, 1977; example item: "I could not 'get going'"), with Cronbach's alphas ranging from .86 to .93 across all waves. Mothers' general mental health symptoms (i.e., somatization, obsessive-compulsive, interpersonal sensitivity, depression, anxiety, hostility, phobic anxiety, paranoid ideation, and psychoticism) were appraised with the 52-item *Brief Symptom Inventory* (Derogatis & Melisaratos, 1983; example item: "Feeling fearful"), with Cronbach's alphas across T1 and T3 varying from 0.94 to 0.96.

Children's adjustment. Caregivers reported children's emotion regulation ability using the 24-item Checklist for Child's Emotion Regulation (Shields & Cicchetti, 1997; example item: "Gets over it quickly when he/she is upset or unhappy"), children's internalizing and externalizing symptoms using the broadband scales of the Child Behavior Checklist (Achenbach & Rescorla, 2001; example item: "Cruelty, bullying, or meanness to others"), and children's social skills using the 33-item Peer Involvement and Social Skills Questionnaire (Walker & McConnell, 1995; example item: "Makes friends easily with other children"). Internalizing problems was the sum of the withdrawn/depressed, anxious/depressed, and somatic complaint scales (32 items) and externalizing problems was the sum of the rule-breaking and aggressive behavior scales (35 items). Cronbach's alpha was 0.87 at T1 and T3 for emotion regulation ability, 0.83–0.92 for internalizing and externalizing symptoms across T1 and T3, and 0.96 at T1 and 0.97 at T3 for social skills.

4.2.6 Analytic Approach

Preliminary analyses were conducted to examine intervention group effects in hair cortisol using repeated-measures analysis of variance (ANOVA) with a within factor of time (T1 vs. T2 or T2 vs. T3) and a between factor of group (intervention vs. comparison). These analyses indicated that there were no significant group differences, $F(1, 31)=0.47$, $p=0.50$ for T1 versus T2 and $F(1, 22)=1.08$, $p=0.31$ for T2 versus T3 and no significant group by time interactions, $F(1, 31)=2.54$, $p=0.12$ and $F(1, 22)=1.62$, $p=0.22$. As a result, subsequent analyses were conducted across intervention and comparison groups.

Mean level differences over time on hair cortisol, parenting stress, emotion dysregulation, and depressive and mental health symptoms were examined using repeated-measures ANOVAs with a within factor of time (in prison comparison T1 vs. T2 or after release comparison T2 vs. T3). Stability over time (in prison: T1 to T2; in prison to after release: T2 to T3) was examined using correlations (one-tail). Associations between mother hair cortisol, mother parenting stress, mother adjustment (i.e., emotion dysregulation and depressive and mental health symptoms), child adjustment (i.e., emotion regulation ability, internalizing and externalizing symptoms, and social skills) and mother-child contact were examined at T1, T2, and T3 using correlations (one-tail) and chi-square analysis.

All cortisol values were recoded to drop values higher than 1,500, indicative of possible contamination, most commonly by hydrocortisone use. Two samples from T1 ($n = 40 - 2 = 38$) and T2 ($n = 36 - 2 = 34$) were dropped because of possible contamination, and no samples were dropped from T3 ($n = 25$). Recoded cortisol variables were further examined and as two T1 and one T3 samples were outliers (>$2SD$ above mean), we recoded them to the next highest value.

4.3 Results

4.3.1 Change Across Time

Hair cortisol. Average levels of mother hair cortisol were compared in prison (T1 vs. T2) and after release (T2 vs. T3; see Table 4.1 for means and standard deviations). Mother hair cortisol did not change when comparing two samples both obtained during stay in prison. However, hair cortisol levels significantly increased from T2 (before release) to T3 (after release), $F(1, 23) = 8.76$, $p < 0.01$.

Parenting stress, emotion dysregulation, and depressive and mental health symptoms. To determine if other aspects changed in similar ways over time to mother hair cortisol, in prison comparisons (T1 vs. T2) and after release comparisons (T2 vs. T3; see Table 4.1 for means and standard deviations) were conducted for other variables. Mother emotion dysregulation significant decreased from T1 (in prison) to T2 (before release), $F(1, 46) = 6.93$, $p < 0.05$, and decreased from T2 (before release) to T3 (after release) at the $p < 0.10$ level, $F(1, 37) = 2.79$, $p < 0.10$. Mother depressive symptoms significantly decreased from T1 to T2, $F(1, 46) = 5.24$, $p < 0.05$, but not

Table 4.1 Means and standard deviations for pairwise comparisons over time

Variable	In prison comparison T1 vs. T2 $N = 47$		Before versus after release comparison T2 vs. T3 $n = 38$	
Mother hair cortisol (ng/g)	225.98	231.79	237.59$_a$	327.58$_b$
	(113.33)	(110.13)	(110.42)	(163.16)
Mother parenting stress	3.00	2.96	3.02	3.20
	(.93)	(.96)	(1.0)	(.96)
Mother emotion dysregulation	72.94$_a$	66.77$_b$	67.18	63.13
	(21.37)	(18.69)	(19.51)	(20.08)
Mother depressive symptoms	17.55$_a$	13.96$_b$	12.66	11.55
	(10.76)	(8.97)	(7.93)	(11.27)
Mother mental health symptoms	.71$_a$	.56$_b$	.54	.56
	(.52)	(.45)	(.44)	(.57)

Note: For hair cortisol, $n = 33$ for the T1 vs. T2 comparison and $n = 24$ for the T2 vs. T3 comparison. Means with different subscripts indicate significant time effects at $p < .05$

from T2 to T3. Similarly, mother mental health symptoms also significantly decreased from T1 to T2, $F(1, 46) = 5.22, p < 0.05$, but not from T2 to T3. For mother parenting stress, there were no significant differences between T1 and T2 or between T2 and T3.

4.3.2 Stability Across Time

Hair cortisol. T1 mother hair cortisol levels in prison were related to T2 hair cortisol levels before release, $r(33) = 0.37, p < 0.05$, and T2 hair cortisol levels before release were related to T3 hair cortisol levels after release, $r(24) = 0.46, p < 0.05$.

Parenting stress, emotion dysregulation, and depressive and mental health symptoms. To determine the stability of other aspects over time in regards to mother hair cortisol, associations in prison (T1 with T2) and after release (T2 with T3) were examined for other variables. T1 mother parenting stress in prison was significantly related to T2 parenting stress before release, $r(47) = 0.73, p < 0.001$, and T2 parenting stress before release was significantly related to T3 parenting stress after release, $r(38) = 0.62, p < 0.001$. T1 mother emotion dysregulation in prison was significantly related to T2 emotion dysregulation before release, $r(47) = 0.69, p < 0.001$, and T2 emotion dysregulation before release was significantly related to T3 emotion dysregulation after release, $r(38) = 0.72, p < 0.001$. T1 mother depressive and mental health symptoms in prison were significantly related to T2 symptoms before release, $r(47) = 0.42, p < 0.01$ and $r(47) = 0.57, p < 0.001$, respectively, and T2 symptoms before release were significantly related to T3 symptoms after release, $r(38) = 0.51, p < 0.001$ and $r(38) = 0.36, p < 0.05$, respectively.

4.3.3 Associations Among Key Constructs

Correlations were conducted to determine associations with mother hair cortisol, mother parenting stress and adjustment (emotion dysregulation, and depressive and mental health symptoms), and children's adjustment (social skills, emotional dysregulation, and internalizing and externalizing symptoms) at each time point. As detailed in the correlation matrix in Table 4.2, mother parenting stress was significantly associated with mother hair cortisol at T1 and T2, and showed a trend association at the $p < 0.10$ level at T3. Mother emotion dysregulation was significantly associated with mother hair cortisol at T1 and associated at the $p < 0.10$ level at T2 and T3. Higher levels of mother parenting stress and mother emotion dysregulation were related to higher levels of hair cortisol. Mother depressive and mental health symptoms were not significantly associated with mother hair cortisol at T1, T2, or T3. Mother emotion dysregulation and mother depressive and mental health symptoms were significantly associated with each other at T1, T2, and T3. Mother parenting stress was also significantly associated with emotion dysregulation at T1, T2,

Table 4.2 Correlations among mother hair cortisol, parenting stress, and adjustment

	Hair cortisol (ng/g)	Parenting stress	Emotion dysregulation	Depressive symptoms	Mental health symptoms
Hair cortisol (ng/g)	–	.40**/.32*	.29*/.23+	.07/–.07	–.05/–.04
Parenting stress	.31+	–	.60***/.58***	.47***/.40**	.33*/.26*
Emotion dysregulation	.29+	.48***	–	.68***/.58***	.46***/.52***
Depressive symptoms	.14	.25+	.71***	–	.82***/.84***
Mental health symptoms	.02	.12	.56**	.89***	–

Note: ***$p<.001$; **$p<.01$; *$p<.05$; +$p<.10$. T1/T2 correlations are above the diagonal, respectively ($N=47$; for T1 hair cortisol, $n=38$, and for T2 hair cortisol, $n=33$). T3 correlations are below the diagonal ($n=38$; for T3 hair cortisol, $n=25$)

Table 4.3 Mother hair cortisol, parenting stress, and adjustment with child adjustment correlations

	Mother hair cortisol (ng/g) T1/T3	Mother parenting stress T1/T3	Mother emotion dysregulation T1/T3	Mother depressive symptoms T1/T3	Mother mental health symptoms T1/T3
Child emotion regulation ability	–.15/–.59**	–.45**/–.50**	–.48**/–.12	–.30*/.04	–.17/.04
Child internalizing	.23/.26	.18/.42*	.52**/.51**	.30*/.26	.18/.24
Child externalizing	.05/41+	.34*/.30+	.32*/.07	.21/–.05	–.03/–.12
Child social skills	–.09/–.32	–.49**/–.32+	–.43**/–.18	–.16/.02	–.07/–.01

Note: ***$p<.001$; **$p<.01$; *$p<.05$; +$p<.10$. At T1, $n=30$; for T1 hair cortisol, $n=24$. At T3, $n=23$; for T3 hair cortisol, $n=15$

and T3, depressive and mental health symptoms at T1 and T2, and associated with depressive symptoms at the $p<0.10$ level at T3.

As shown in the correlation matrix in Table 4.3, at T1, mother parenting stress was significantly related to child difficulty regulating emotions, externalizing symptoms, and poor social skills. Mothers' emotion dysregulation was significantly related to child difficulty regulating emotions, internalizing and externalizing symptoms, and poor social skills. Mothers' depressive symptoms were significantly related to child difficulty regulating emotions and internalizing symptoms. At T3, mothers' higher hair cortisol was significantly related to child difficulty regulating emotions. Similar to T1, at T3, higher mother parenting stress was significantly related to child difficulty regulating emotions and internalizing symptoms and related to child externalizing and poor social skills at the $p<0.10$ level. Also at T3, mothers' greater emotion dysregulation was significantly related to child internalizing symptoms.

4.3.4 Associations with Mother–Child Contact

Correlations between mother-child contact (living with child full or part time before incarceration, frequency of in-person or telephone contact in past month or after release, length of time since last in-person visit, telephone call, or contact by letter, living with child full or part time after release) and mother hair cortisol, parenting stress, adjustment, and child adjustment were examined at each time point. In addition, correlations with time incarcerated were examined at each time point and correlations with recidivism as indicated by being detained in the 6 months after release. As detailed in the correlation matrix in Table 4.4, living with their child before incarceration was significantly associated with lower levels of hair cortisol at T1 in prison and living with their child after release was associated at the $p<0.10$ level with lower levels of hair cortisol at T3. Follow up ANOVAs to examine mean level differences revealed that mothers who lived with their child before incarceration had significantly lower levels of hair cortisol at T1 in prison ($M=193.20$, $SD=90.32$) compared to mothers who did not live with their child ($M=323.52$, $SD=134.72$), $F(1, 37)=11.24$, $p<0.01$ (but not at T2 before release or T3 after release). However, mothers who lived with their child after incarceration did not have significantly lower levels of hair cortisol at T3 after release ($M=273.22$, $SD=157.59$) compared to mothers who did not live with their child ($M=358.85$, $SD=162.53$), $F(1, 24)=1.76$, $p=0.20$.

Longer length of time since last contact was significantly associated with higher levels of hair cortisol at T1 in prison only. Time incarcerated was associated at the $p<0.10$ level with hair cortisol at T3 after release (see Table 4.4). The longer women were in prison, the higher their post-release cortisol levels. Longer time incarcerated was also significantly associated with higher levels of mother mental health symptoms at T1 in prison and T2 before release but not at T3 after release. Frequency of contact in past month was not related to hair cortisol at T1 in prison or T2 before release, and frequency of contact since release was not related to hair cortisol at T3 after release.

In regards to children (see Table 4.4), none of the child adjustment variables significantly related to whether mothers lived with their children before or after release. There was a significant association between frequency of contact between mothers and children and children's internalizing symptoms at T1. The more frequent the contact between mothers and children, the greater children's internalizing symptoms at T1. Mothers' time incarcerated was significantly related to children's emotion regulation difficulties and poor social skills at T1 and T3 and children's

4 Associations Among Mother–Child Contact, Parenting Stress, and Mother... 73

Table 4.4 Correlations with mother-child contact

	Lived with child before incarceration (1=yes, 0=no) T1	T2	T3	Frequency of contact (in-person or phone) in last month or since release T1	T2	T3	Length of time since last contact (in-person, phone, or letter) T1	T2	T3	Time incarcerated T1	T2	T3	Lived with child after release (1=yes, 0=no) T3
Mothers													
Hair cortisol (ng/g)	−.49***	−.15	−.15	−.14	.21	−.04	.30*	.15	.12	.01	−.12	.32⁺	−.27⁺
Parenting stress	−.10	.03	.07	.05	.11	.26⁺	−.06	.06	−.49***	.27*	.16	.25⁺	.06
Emotion dysregulation	−.09	.05	.12	.02	.11	.02	.02	−.16	−.07	.10	−.02	−.06	−.13
Depressive symptoms	.09	.02	−.07	−.09	.04	−.14	.01	−.13	.05	.15	.20⁺	−.19	−.09
Mental health symptoms	.11	.00	−.18	−.01	.05	−.22	.12	−.04	.13	.24*	.39**	−.13	−.16
Detention (1=yes, 0=no)			−.42**			−.38**			.04			−.29*	−.44**
Children													
Emotion regulation ability	.02			−.28⁺		−.15	.12		.14	−.39*		−.47**	.01
Internalizing	.05			.38*		.29⁺	−.28⁺		−.25	.001		.31⁺	.19
Externalizing	.08			.08		.14	−.03		−.10	.04		.50**	−.02
Social skills	−.07			−.21		−.12	.13		.11	−.49**		−.40*	.13

Note: ****p*<.001; ***p*<.01; **p*<.05; ⁺*p*<.10. For mothers: *N*=47 at T1 and T2 and *n*=38 at T3. For children: *N*=30 at T1 and *n*=23 at T3. For hair cortisol, *n*=38 at T1, *n*=33 at T2, and *n*=25 at T3

externalizing at T3. The longer mothers were incarcerated, the lower children's abilities to regulate their emotions and social skills were at both T1 and T3 and the greater children's externalizing symptoms at T3.

Associations between recidivism and mother-child contact indicated that mother' living with child before incarceration, more frequent contact while in prison, and living with child after release were significantly associated with less recidivism (see Table 4.4). Lower recidivism also was related to longer incarceration times. Follow up ANOVAs to examine mean level differences indicated that mothers who were detained in the 6 months after release had significantly less contact with their child ($M=2.00$, $SD=2.00$) compared to mothers who were not detained ($M=3.93$, $SD=1.84$), $F(1, 37)=6.06$, $p<0.05$. For time incarcerated, the group difference approached significance at the $p<.10$ level. Mothers who were detained by T3 had spent less time (in months) incarcerated ($M=22.26$, $SD=14.03$) compared to mothers who were not detained after release ($M=38.12$, $SD=23.25$), $F(1, 37)=3.35$, $p<0.10$. Whether mothers were detained post-release was significantly associated with living with their child before incarceration, χ^2 ($n=38$, $df=1$) $=6.84$, $p<0.01$, and after release, χ^2 ($n=38$, $df=1$) $=7.37$, $p<0.01$. Of the mothers who were detained after release, 63 % did not live with their child before incarceration and 100 % did not live with their child after release. In contrast, of the mothers who were not detained after release, 83 % lived with their child before incarceration and 63 % lived with their child after release.

4.4 Discussion

The present study was intended as a first step toward illuminating pathways linking stressors, parent stress (biological and psychosocial, including that related to parenting), and parent and child adjustment during the period of time before and after incarcerated parents are released from prison. This transitional period may be critical to the future adjustment of both mother and child (Travis & Waul, 2003), and learning more about the psychological and social processes in play during this time is vital to developing effective preventive interventions that improve short and long term outcomes for mothers, children, and families. We now discuss the implications of our findings.

4.4.1 Mother–Child Contact

Findings were mixed in regards to the association between mother-child contact and indices of maternal and child adjustment. At T1 in prison, mother-child contact may have served as a maternal stress buffer, with lower cortisol levels detected among mothers who had lived with their child prior to incarceration and who, while in prison, had been in more recent contact with their child. For children, however, more contact (as defined as frequency of visits or phone calls) with incarcerated mothers was related to higher child internalizing symptoms. In contrast, longer periods of mother incarceration, and thus more limited contact between mother and child, were related not only to children's emotion regulation difficulties and poorer social skills, but also to child externalizing behaviors. Both findings suggest the need for careful consideration of contact, and lack thereof, by parents and caregivers, service providers, and corrections and other related public systems.

In terms of the first finding, this is not the first study to find negative effects related to contact between incarcerated parents and children (see Poehlmann et al., 2010), and this finding raises questions regarding not only why some children had more internalizing symptoms related to more frequent contact and other children do not, but also what might be done to buffer this potentially problematic outcome. Particularly important issues to consider include what a child has been told about his or her mother's situation, how a child is prepared for a call or visit by his or her caregivers and his or her mother, what mothers and caregivers and prison staff do to help calls and visits go well, and how both caregiver and mother interact with the child after a call or a visit.

In terms of the second finding, as noted elsewhere in this paper and in this monograph, prison time can be stressful on all family members, including children. One of the most consistent findings in the literature is that the children of incarcerated parents are at elevated risk for exhibiting externalizing behaviors (Murray et al., 2012), and problems with emotion regulation and poor social skills could be considered be part of a constellation of more serious problems of child conduct (e.g., Oppositional Defiant Disorder, Conduct Disorder) or correlates of such problems. Externalizing behavior may be one response to this stress. However, the story may be more complicated. For example, the relation between longer sentences (and thus reduced mother-child contact) and increased externalizing problems for children may be due primarily to reverberations from the incarceration, including separation from parent, and/or due to a combination of this and problems present before the incarceration, such as exposure to parent criminality and its correlates, such as increased exposure to delinquent peers, reduced parental supervision and monitoring, and increased inept discipline. Regardless, the relation between sentence length and child problems points to the challenges of parenting a child with a mother in prison, and the need for support for the parent/caregiver who is parenting the child on the outside.

In recent years, advocates have declared a "bill of rights" for children of incarcerated parents, with the most attention paid to the "right to speak with, see and touch my parent" (San Francisco Partnership for Incarcerated Parents, 2003b). No less important in this bill is the "right to support as I struggle with my parent's incarceration". An appropriate companion to the bill would be a statement of the responsibilities of all concerned to prepare, guide, and comfort a child through the process of contact, and lack of contact, with an incarcerated parent.

In terms of research, future investigations of mother-child contact might explore how to increase the quality of various types of mother-child communication (whether face-to-face, on the phone, or via letter), such as how contexts might be changed to enhance in person visitation. Rigorous trials of parenting interventions, including visitation interventions, for both incarcerated mothers and for parents and other caregivers in the community are very much needed to inform the field on "best" practices and policies relevant to incarcerated mothers and their families.

4.4.2 Maternal Stress and Adjustment

Maternal cortisol values remained stable while mothers were in prison, and increased significantly after release. This pattern of cortisol change following release from prison is unique in comparison with the trajectories of other key constructs over time. Mothers' self-reported parenting stress remained stable over the three time points, while mothers' emotion dysregulation showed a linear decreasing trend, and both depression and other mental health symptoms fell while mothers were still in prison and remained stable after release. Across all three waves, higher maternal cortisol related to higher levels of parenting stress and emotion dysregulation. It was somewhat surprising, given the neurochemistry of depression that closely hews to the HPA axis, that cortisol was not significantly correlated with depressive and mental health symptoms at any wave. That parenting stress and emotion dysregulation post-release did not spike in tandem with maternal cortisol suggests that mothers' high physiological stress levels may have been responsive to factors, whether stressful or not, that were not captured here, such as securing employment and housing, and negotiating relationships apart from those with children (Travis & Waul, 2003).

Of interest in terms of future research, self-report and biological measures of stress provided unique information regarding relations among mother-child contact, and mother and child outcomes. While the average cortisol levels reflecting incarcerated mothers' stress at three distinct time points before release (T1), before release but after the *Emotions Program* (T2), and within six months of release from prison (T3) appear to be high, it will be important to determine in future research whether cortisol values for incarcerated mothers are higher than values reported in prior studies of non-incarcerated populations (e.g., Thomson et al., 2010). As is already evident in numerous other studies (see Haney, 2003), incarceration can be a stressful experience. The period after release also appears to be stressful physiologically. Given these findings, incarcerated mothers, their children, and family members, may be in a position to benefit from effective stress management techniques to help them cope both with the incarceration period as well as during the transition home.

It is unclear why associations between greater mother-child contact and lower maternal stress at T1 did not hold up at T2 just prior to mothers' release. However, this period is one of a new type of stress, marked by heightened anticipation and hope. It may be that the three time points examined here present three very different psychological and environmental "settings" in which to examine the relations among these variables.

Research based on self-report measures indicates that mother and child stress can surge during reunification (Cobbina & Bender, 2012), and mothers' cortisol values at T3, the highest recorded during this study, provide additional support for this phenomenon, especially as hair cortisol levels were compared to participants' own baseline levels obtained during imprisonment. Surprisingly, at T3, maternal cortisol levels did not relate to mother-child contact in the form of living together, frequency of contact, and duration since last contact with their child. Similarly, these measures of mother-child contact did not significantly relate to children's adjustment. Instead, at T3, most indicators of child functioning were sensitive to mothers' stress, with parenting stress relating to children's difficulties regulating their emotions and to higher internalizing symptoms, and higher maternal cortisol levels post-release relating to children's poorer emotion regulation. Though mothers' emotion dysregulation at T3 was significantly associated with higher children's internalizing symptoms, this was the only finding post-release linking maternal adjustment to child adjustment. In all, the evidence pointed to the role of maternal stress as a proximal influence on children's adjustment post-release.

Given the constellation of other potential stressors that women may experience post-release (Travis & Waul, 2003), it is possible that the earlier positive influence on mothers' cortisol of closer contact with children may be overwhelmed by the acute stressors associated with readjustment to life outside prison. Stressors associated with readjustment may have been more acute for some women than for others; the finding that women with longer sentences had higher cortisol levels raises questions of whether these women experienced more intense prisonization that may have rendered them particularly vulnerable to the impact of stressors associated with community readjustment. Longer prison sentences and/or their precursors and consequences may be disabling for children, too; at T3, the children of women who served longer sentences were at greater risk of poor outcomes across every child variable measured.

Somewhat complex relations among cortisol, parenting stress, and mother-child contact emerged at T3 that may have implications for supports for incarcerated mothers post-release. While mothers were in prison (at T1 and T2), mother-child contact was unrelated to self-reported parenting stress; it was not until mothers were released that increased contact with children related to higher self-reported parenting stress. Higher parenting stress, in turn, was related to elevated cortisol. It is possible that an indirect relationship exists between mother-child contact and cortisol through changes in parenting stress, a hypothesis that would need to be tested with a larger sample. Though mother-child contact also appears to be protective as suggested by reduced recidivism rates among mothers who had more frequent contact and lived with their children before and after incarceration, engaged parenting on the outside may also serve as a unique stressor for newly released mothers—with potentially direct implications for mothers' psychosocial stress and indirect effects for physiological stress—that warrants further investigation.

The findings regarding cortisol and the potentially debilitating effects of longer sentences raise several questions of relevance to the healthy adjustment of children of incarcerated parents. As discussed above, one of the most proximal influences on healthy child adjustment is effective parenting. Effective parenting includes the consistent practice of positive parenting skills while remaining physically and emotionally present with children, which may be deleteriously affected by depression, emotion dysregulation, and other forms of poor parent adjustment. In the present study, strengthening incarcerated mothers' adjustment has implications for mothers' being able to parent well, with clear benefits for children. Despite our identification of the highest levels of positive maternal adjustment at T3, average maternal cortisol was also at its highest point in the study. This finding suggests that stress may exert effects—unique from those related to maternal adjustment—on formerly incarcerated mothers and their children.

It remains unclear, however, which stress-related elements may place certain former inmates and, by extension, their children, at heightened risk. Are former prisoners at greater risk for difficult reunification if they have greater stress responsiveness post-release as reflected in cortisol spikes that may have remained consistently elevated, have particularly poor coping responses, and/or did individual experiences and perceptions of stressors play a role? It is possible that all of these phenomena occur simultaneously, for instance, with high cortisol potentially impairing women's capacities to exercise sound judgment, and women coping with stress in ways that are no longer adaptive (e.g., social isolation). Women's individual perceptions, often honed in response to a lifetime of adversity, may have played a role; one former incarcerated mother might perceive of a stressor as meddlesome while another might perceive of the same phenomenon as traumatic and highly stressful. Further, former incarcerated mothers may have been exposed to different stressors depending on the legacy they bring with them based on issues such as their specific crimes, the social relationships they return to, and how they are influenced by their past, and how long they were imprisoned and the impact this has on their mental functioning (Haney, 2003). Finally, in many states, women who served time for felony drug convictions are ineligible for public assistance and certain types of employment (San Francisco Partnership for Incarcerated Parents, 2003). Issues such as these may contribute to more stress for some women than for others.

4.4.3 Recidivism

The implications of mother-child contact for recidivism after prison release are emphasized by the study's findings. Mothers who lived with their child before incarceration, had more frequent contact after release, served more prison time, and lived with their child after release were less likely to get in trouble with the police and be detained in the six months after release. Given these relations, interventions with mothers and caregivers during prison designed to improve communication and begin to bring healing to often strained relationships seem of particular interest. Such work has the potential to assist mothers in rebuilding and strengthening support systems that provide much needed buffers both during prison and after release. Further, interventions designed to improve parent–child relationships and parenting skills also seem warranted. If findings identified here are replicated with larger samples, it may be that intervention efforts focused on positive family and social bonds may have immediate and long term impacts in lowered recidivism as well as more healthy maternal and child adjustment.

4.4.4 Limitations

A key limitation to the present study is the small sample size, and related issues, such as the lack of adequate representation of various racial and ethnic groups in the sample. Clearly, this study is just a first step to examining the issues discussed here, and additional work is required with larger and more representative samples. In addition, for various reasons, including religious beliefs, assessors encountered sensitivity among incarcerated women related to the collection of hair as a biological sample, and some women opted out of this component of the study, leading to missing data. As a counter to this, staff inserted into the standard Van Uum hair protocol several additional check-ins with participants regarding their level of comfort with each step of the protocol. This approach, combined with the strong rapport developed between study assessors and many mothers over the course of this longitudinal study, led to many participants agreeing to donate a hair sample at T3. It is possible that some hair samples were influenced by hydrocortisone as some women reported receiving unlabeled prescription creams from prison health providers and not knowing what they contained. Cortisol values indicative of possible contamination were recoded prior to analysis as previously noted.

4.5 Conclusion

The present study sought to identify areas of vulnerability that might be shored up prior to release and during the post-release process of reintegration back into day-to-day life in the community. For many mothers, this means once again becoming the primary caregiver. An important candidate during this period appears to be maternal stress, which may serve as a key proximal influence on children's adjustment post-release. If this finding holds up in future studies, this result implies that one avenue for promoting positive readjustment for formerly incarcerated mothers and their children involves helping mothers to effectively reduce their psychosocial and physiological stress and related negative coping. By supporting mothers' abilities to manage stress while promoting mothers' positive parenting skills and healthy adjustment, mothers' abilities to parent effectively may be safeguarded, along with their children's overall well-being. A second, synergistic, candidate appears to be mother-child contact while mothers are incarcerated. By supporting both mothers and their children as they do, and do not have contact, stress may be reduced and well-being may be promoted. Rigorous basic and intervention research is needed on these topics so that a knowledge base is available to better guide families—and the professionals who serve them—as they struggle with the challenges of incarceration and its aftermath.

Acknowledgements We thank the mothers and their families and the Oregon Department of Corrections and the Coffee Creek Correctional Facility and their staff members for their participation in this study. Work on this manuscript was supported by the primary grant for this study, Award R34 MH 79911 from the United States Department of Health and Human Services, National Institutes of Health (NIH), National Institute of Mental Health (NIMH), as well as by Award 90CA178/1/04 from the United States Department of Health and Human Services, Administration for Children and Families (ACF), Children's Bureau, Office of Child Abuse and Neglect. The content is solely the responsibility of the authors and does not necessarily represent the official views of the NIH, the NIMH, or the ACF.

References

Achenbach, T. M., & Rescorla, L. A. (2001). *Manual for ASEBA school-age forms and profiles*. Burlington, VT: University of Vermont, Research Center for Children, Youth, and Families.

Bales, W. D., & Mears, D. P. (2008). Inmate social ties and the transition to society: Does visitation reduce recidivism? *Journal of Research in Crime and Delinquency, 45*, 287–321. doi:10.1177/0022427808317574.

Carlson, J. R. (1998). Evaluating the effectiveness of a live-in nursery within a women's prison. *Journal of Offender Rehabilitation, 27*, 73–85. doi:10.1300/J076v27n01_06.

Cobbina, J. E., & Bender, K. A. (2012). Predicting the future: Incarcerated women's views of reentry success. *Journal of Offender Rehabilitation, 51*, 275–294. doi:10.1080/10509674.2012.683323.

Derogatis, L. R., & Melisaratos, N. (1983). The brief symptom inventory: An introductory report. *Psychological Medicine, 13*, 595–605. doi:10.1017/S0033291700048017.

Dettenborn, L., Tietze, A., Bruckner, F., & Kirschbaum, C. (2010). Higher cortisol content in hair among long-term unemployed individuals compared to controls. *Psychoneuroendocrinology, 35*, 1404–1409. doi:10.1016/j.psyneuen.2010.04.006.

Eddy, J. M., Kjellstrand, J., Martinez, C. R., Jr., & Newton, R. (2010). Theory-based multimodal parenting intervention for incarcerated parents and their families. In J. M. Eddy & J. Poehlmann (Eds.), *Children of incarcerated parents: A handbook for researchers and practitioners* (pp. 237–261). Washington, DC: The Urban Institute.

Eddy, J. M., Martinez, C. R., Jr., Schiffmann, T., Newton, R., Olin, L., Leve, L., et al. (2008). Development of a multisystemic parent management training intervention for incarcerated parents, their children and families. *Clinical Psychologist, 12*, 86–98. doi:10.1080/13284200802495461.

Eddy, J. M., Martinez, C. R., Jr., & Burraston, B. (2013). A randomized controlled trial of a parent management training program for incarcerated parents: Proximal impacts. In J. Eddy & J. M. Poehlmann (Eds.), *Children of incarcerated parents: Multidisciplinary perspectives on research, intervention, and policy* (pp. 108–134). Washington, DC: Urban Institute.

Gibbons, F. X., Etcheverry, P. E., Stock, M. L., Gerrard, M., Weng, C., Kiviniemi, M., et al. (2010). Exploring the link between racial discrimination and substance use: What mediates? What buffers? *Journal of Personality and Social Psychology, 99*, 785–801. doi:10.1037/a0019880.

Gibbons, F. X., Gerrard, M., Cleveland, M. J., Wills, T. A., & Brody, G. H. (2004). Perceived discrimination and substance use in African American parents and their children: A panel study. *Journal of Personality and Social Psychology, 86*, 517–529. doi:10.1037/0022-3514.86.4.517.

Glaze, L. E., & Maruschak, L. M. (2008). Parents in prison and their minor children (NCJ 222984). Washington, DC: United States Department of Justice, Office of Justice Programs, Bureau of Justice Statistics. Retrieved from http://bjs.gov/content/pub/pdf/pptmc.pdf

Gratz, K. L., & Roemer, L. (2004). Multidimensional assessment of emotion regulation and dysregulation: Development, factor structure, and initial validation of the difficulties in emotion regulation scale. *Journal of Psychopathology and Behavioral Assessment, 26*, 41–54. doi:10.1023/B:JOBA.0000007455.08539.94.

Greenfield, L., & Snell, T. (2000). *Women offenders* (NCJ 175688). Washington, DC: United States Department of Justice, Office of Justice Programs, Bureau of Justice Statistics. Retrieved from http://www.bjs.gov/content/pub/pdf/wo.pdf

Gunnar, M. R., & Donzella, B. (2002). Social regulation of the cortisol levels in early human development. *Psychoneuroendocrinology, 27*, 199–220. doi:10.1016/S0306-4530(01)00045-2.

Gunnar, M. R., & Vazquez, D. M. (2001). Low cortisol and a flattening of expected daytime rhythm: Potential indices of risk in human development. *Developmental Psychopathology, 13*, 515–538. doi:10.1017/S0954579401003066.

Hagan, J., & Coleman, J. P. (2001). Returning captives of the American war on drugs: Issues of community and family reentry. *Crime and Delinquency, 47*, 352–367. doi:10.1177/0011128701047003004.

Haney, C. (2003). The psychological impact of incarceration: Implications for postprison adjustment. In J. Travis & M. Waul (Eds.), *The impact of incarceration and reentry on children, families, and communities* (pp. 33–66). Washington, DC: The Urban Institute.

Hellhammer, D. H., Wüst, S., & Kudielka, B. M. (2009). Salivary cortisol as a biomarker in stress research. *Psychoneuroendocrinology, 34*, 163–171. doi:10.1016/j.psyneuen.2008.10.026.

Herman, J. (1992). A new diagnosis. In J. Herman (Ed.), *Trauma and recovery* (pp. 115–132). New York: Basic Books.

Holt, N., & Miller, D. (1972). *Explorations in inmate-family relationships* (Research Report No. 46). Sacramento, CA: California Department of Corrections.

Kalra, S., Einarson, A., Karskov, T., Van Uum, S., & Koren, G. (2007). The relationship between stress and hair cortisol in healthy pregnant women. *Clinical and Investigative Medicine, 30*, E103–E107.

Kjellstrand, J. M., Cearley, J., Eddy, J. M., Foney, D., & Martinez, C. R., Jr. (2012). Characteristics of incarcerated fathers and mothers: Implications for preventive interventions targeting children and families. *Children and Youth Services Review, 34*, 2409–2415. doi:10.1016/j.childyouth.2012.08.008.

Kjellstrand, J. M., & Eddy, J. M. (2011a). Parental incarceration during childhood, family context, and youth problem behavior across adolescence. *Journal of Offender Rehabilitation, 50*, 18–36. doi:10.1080/10509674.2011.536720.

Kjellstrand, J. M., & Eddy, J. M. (2011b). Mediators of the effect of parental incarceration on adolescent externalizing behaviors. *Journal of Community Psychology, 39*, 551–565. doi:10.1002/jcop.20451.

Masten, A., & Garmezy, N. (1985). Risk, vulnerability, and protective factors in developmental psychopathology. In B. Lahey & A. Kazdin (Eds.), *Advances in clinical child psychology* (pp. 1–52). New York: Plenum.

McEwen, B. S., & Wingfield, J. (2003). The concept of allostatis in biology and biomedicine. *Hormones and Behavior, 43*, 2–15. doi:10.1016/S0018-506X(02)00024-7.

McMahon, R. J., & Lengua, L. (1996). *Being a parent* (Technical Report) [On-line]. Retrieved from http://www.fasttrackproject.org/

Minnesota Department of Corrections. (2011). *The effects of prison visitation on offender recidivism* (Research Report). St. Paul, MN. Retrieved from http://www.doc.state.mn.us/pages/files/large-files/Publications/11-11MNPrisonVisitationStudy.pdf

Murray, J., Farrington, D. P., & Sekol, I. (2012). Children's antisocial behavior, mental health, drug use, and educational performance after parental incarceration: A systematic review and meta-analysis. *Psychological Bulletin, 138*, 175–210. doi:10.1037/a0026407.

Peat, B., & Winfree, T. (1992). Reducing the intra-institutional effects of 'prisonization': A study of a therapeutic community for drug-using inmates. *Criminal Justice and Behavior, 19*, 206–225. doi:10.1177/0093854892019002007.

Pereg, D., Gow, R., Mosseri, M., Lishner, M., Rieder, M., Van Uum, S., et al. (2010). Hair cortisol and the risk for acute myocardial infarction in adult men. *Stress, 14*, 73–81. doi:10.1037/a0026407.

Poehlmann, J. (2005). Incarcerated mother's contact with children, perceived family relationships, and depressive symptoms. *Journal of Family Psychology, 19*, 350–357. doi:10.1037/0893-3200.19.3.350.

Poehlmann, J., Dallaire, D., Loper, A. B., & Shear, L. D. (2010). Children's contact with their incarcerated parents: Research findings and recommendations. *American Psychologist, 65*, 575–598. doi:10.1037/a0020279.

Poehlmann, J., & Eddy, J. M. (Eds.) (2013). *Relationship processes and resilience in children with incarcerated parents*. Monographs of the Society for Research in Child Development, Serial No. 308. Chichester: Wiley.

Radloff, L. S. (1977). The CES-D scale: A self-report depression scale for research in the general population. *Applied Psychological Measurement, 1*, 385–401. doi:10.1177/014662167700100306.

Rosmond, R. (2001). Visceral obesity and the metabolic syndrome. In P. Björntorp (Ed.), *The international textbook of obesity* (pp. 339–350). Chichester: Wiley.

Russell, E., Koren, G., Rieder, M., & Van Uum, S. (2012). Hair cortisol as a biological marker of chronic stress: Current status, future directions and unanswered questions. *Psychoneuroendocrinology, 37*, 589–601. doi:10.1016/j.psyneuen.2011.09.009.

San Francisco Partnership for Incarcerated Parents. (2003a). *Panel discussion on the rights and needs of the children of incarcerated parents*. San Francisco, CA.

San Francisco Partnership for Incarcerated Parents (2003b). *Children of incarcerated parents: A bill of rights*. San Franciso, CA.

Sapolsky, R. M. (2004). Social status and health in humans and other animals. *Annual Review of Anthropology, 33*, 393–418. doi:10.1146/annurev.anthro.33.070203.144000.

Sapolsky, R. M., Romero, L. M., & Munck, A. U. (2000). How do glucocorticoids influence stress responses? Integrating permissive, suppressive, stimulatory, and preparative actions. *Endocrine Reviews, 21*, 55–89.

Schiffmann, T. J., Eddy, J. M., Martinez, C. R., Jr., Leve, L., & Newton, R. (2008). *Parenting inside out: Parent management training for incarcerated parents in prison*. Portland, OR: Oregon Social Learning Center and Children's Justice Alliance.

Shields, A., & Cicchetti, D. (1997). Emotion regulation among school-age children: The development and validation of a new criterion Q-sort scale. *Developmental Psychology, 33*, 906–916. doi:10.1037/0012-1649.33.6.906.

Shortt, J. W., Eddy, J. M., Sheeber, L., & Davis, B. (2014). Project Home: A pilot evaluation of an emotion-focused intervention for mothers reuniting with children after prison. *Psychological Services, 11*, 1–9. doi:10.1037/a0034323.

Steudte, S., Stalder, T., Dettenborn, L., Klumbies, E., Foley, P., Beesdo-Baum, K., et al. (2011). Decreased hair cortisol concentrations in generalised anxiety disorder. *Psychiatry Research, 186*, 310–314. doi:10.1016/j.psychres.2010.09.002.

Thomson, S., Koren, G., Fraser, L. A., Rieder, M., Friedman, T. C., & Van Uum, S. H. M. (2010). Hair analysis provides a historical record of cortisol levels in Cushing's syndrome. *Experimental and Clinical Endocrinology and Diabetes, 118*, 133–138. doi:10.1055/s-0029-1220771.

Travis, J., & Waul, M. (Eds.). (2003). *The impact of incarceration and reentry on children, families, and communities*. Washington, DC: The Urban Institute.

Van Uum, S. H., Sauve, B., Fraser, L. A., Morley-Forster, P., Paul, T. L., & Koren, G. (2008). Elevated content of cortisol in hair of patients with severe chronic pain: A novel biomarker for stress. *Stress, 11*, 483–488. doi:10.1080/10253890801887388.

Walker, H. M., & McConnell, S. (1995). *The Walker-McConnell scale of social competence and school adjustment*. Austin, TX: Pro-Ed.

West, H. C., & Sabol, W. (2008). *Prisoners in 2007* (NCJ 224280). Washington, DC: United States Department of Justice, Office of Justice Programs, Bureau of Justice Statistics. Retrieved from http://www.bjs.gov/content/pub/pdf/p07.pdf

Williams, D. R., & Mohammed, S. A. (2009). Discrimination and racial disparities in health: Evidence and needed research. *Journal of Behavioral Medicine, 32*, 20–47. doi:10.1007/s10865-008-9185-0.

Yamada, J., Stevens, B., de Silva, N., Gibbins, S., Beyene, J., Taddio, A., et al. (2007). Hair cortisol as a potential biologic marker of chronic stress in hospitalized neonates. *Neonatology, 92*, 42–49. doi:10.1159/000100085.

Chapter 5
Children's Contact with Incarcerated Parents: Summary and Recommendations

Julie Poehlmann-Tynan

One in 28 children in the United States has a parent behind bars (The Pew Charitable Trusts, 2010) and even more children are affected if one examines risk for having an incarcerated parent across childhood (Wildeman & Western, 2010). Given these statistics, it is not surprising that children are common visitors in corrections facilities, at prisons and jails. For example, in the 12-month period between July 2011 and June 2012, the Wisconsin Department of Corrections recorded visits at half of their adult male corrections facilities and found that 48,000 visits from children occurred, with more than 131 children walking into Wisconsin state prison visiting rooms per day. Although similar data are not available for local jails, previous research suggests that families may more likely to visit loved ones in local jails than prisons, in part because of the location of jails is typically in closer proximity to where inmates' families live (Arditti, Lambert-Shute, & Joest, 2003).

Recent research has shown that children of incarcerated parents are more likely to exhibit trauma symptoms than other children, but that the link between parental incarceration and child trauma symptoms may be mediated through the quality of parental visitation experiences (Arditti & Savla, 2013). These findings emphasize the importance of not only visit frequency but also of visit quality for children with incarcerated parents. Because children are frequent visitors to corrections facilities and the experiences can be emotionally intense for children and their family members, it is important to examine policies, procedures, and interventions that might improve the experience of visitation and other forms of contact for this vulnerable group of children.

In the summary of this monograph, I first discuss important considerations when examining parent–child contact and delineate several methodological contributions of the papers in this volume. I then offer suggestions relating to changes in policies, procedures,

---

J. Poehlmann-Tynan, Ph.D. (✉)
Human Development & Family Studies, University of Wisconsin-Madison,
1300 Linden Drive, Madison, WI 53706, USA
e-mail: poehlmann@waisman.wisc.edu

and practices that may improve the experience of parent–child contact during parental incarceration as well as fostering the well-being of affected children and families. Some critics may consider these suggestions premature, based on data that need rigorous replication, and I agree. But I also agree with Kurt Lewin, a pioneering social psychologist, who stated, "If you want truly to understand something, try to change it."

5.1 Considerations When Examining Parent–Child Contact in the Context of Parental Incarceration

The introduction to this volume (Shlafer, Loper, & Schillmoeller, 2015), as well as previous research (Poehlmann, Dallaire, Loper, & Shear, 2010), indicates that the type of institutional setting is an important determinant of what types of contact between incarcerated individuals and their family members are allowed or encouraged. Whereas the majority of state and federal prisons offer face-to-face visits (whether these occur across a table or in a more child-friendly setting with toys), most locally-operated jails offer barrier or video visitation rather than face-to-face visits. Because visitation procedures can vary across institutions within the same corrections system, Shlafer et al. (2015) collected data on the type of visits offered at the largest prison in each state. They found that information about visitation and other forms of contact may be difficult for family members and professionals to locate, as some information is not listed on websites and some facilities do not provide information about visit logistics over the phone unless the caller is already on the inmate's visit list.

Time allowed for visits varies widely across institutional settings as well, ranging from 15 min visits to extended visits, and wait times vary substantially. Security procedures differ across institutions, and these procedures may impact children's proximal experiences of different forms of visitation (e.g., video versus barrier visits). In addition to variations in visits, the frequency of telephone calls allowed, privacy offered during calls, and cost associated with phone usage vary from corrections facility to facility as well. Family considerations such as children's age, preparation and support provided by caregivers, and family resources available for transportation and telephone calls vary across families. The complexity of and variation in all of these factors can make it difficult to systematically study parent–child contact across different correctional institutions and different families.

5.2 Methodological Contributions of Monograph

Although contact between parents and children during incarceration may be important for the well-being of both children and parents, findings have been not entirely consistent across studies. Moreover, most studies of parent–child contact in the context of parental incarceration have been conducted using data from one timepoint, and studies have almost exclusively relied upon reports of frequency or type of contact rather than quality, with a few exceptions (e.g., Arditti & Savla, 2013). Although personal visits have been occasionally studied separately from letter-writing and telephone calls, many studies have combined these types of contact. Prison and jail samples are often combined (e.g., Fragile Families and Child Wellbeing Study; Murray, Farrington, & Sekol, 2012) and family, relational, and physiological processes potentially linking the experience of parental incarceration with children's and incarcerated parents' outcomes have rarely been examined (Eddy & Poehlmann, 2010; Poehlmann & Eddy, 2013).

In this monograph, new studies are presented that address some, but not all, of these limitations. Two of the studies focused on jail samples and one focused on a prison sample. Children's age ranges were specified and narrower than in some previous studies and measures of child functioning were developmentally appropriate. Innovative multi-method approaches were employed across the studies, including reliance on multiple reporters of children's behaviors, observational methods, and analysis of physiological stress processes. Moreover, the McClure et al. (2015) study presented longitudinal data, following families into the reunification period. Dallaire, Zeman, and Thrash (2015) analyzed letter-writing and telephone calls separately from personal visits, although McClure et al. did not, and Poehlmann-Tynan et al. (2015) further examined the processes that occur during different types of visits.

Because of their relatively large sample size, Dallaire et al. (2015) were able to test a structural equation model, which indicated a better fit for combining alternate forms of contact (letter-writing and telephone calls) yet separating them from visits. The relation between parent–child contact and child behavior problems varied as a function of type of contact, underscoring the importance of their modeling procedures. This result is not surprising, as children's proximal experiences of in-person barrier visits vastly differ from their experiences talking with a parent on the telephone or reading and writing letters. To further understand the processes that occur during barrier visits and other non-contact visitation procedures, Poehlmann-Tynan et al. (2015) used observational methods in the jail setting. The study highlighted the importance of child-caregiver relationships and supports for young children during the visit process, as well as the tendency for children to become more behaviorally dysregulated during non-contact visits compared to their home environments. Use of observational methods in corrections settings is unique and can help us understand how children react to aspects of visitation, including security and screening procedures, waiting in the corrections setting, and visiting with parents. Although some authors have suggested that certain experiences that occur during visits with parents in corrections facilities may be difficult or even traumatizing for children, few data have been available to verify or refute these speculations. Yet because the study relied on a small sample and used innovative, newly-developed methods, replication is needed, especially for wider age groups.

McClure et al. (2015) presented longitudinal data about contact and maternal adjustment at three timepoints, including data after the mother's release from prison. Following families during the reunification period is a rarity in the literature focusing on parental incarceration and an important step in documenting the longer-term implications of parent–child contact for maternal and family functioning. Importantly, more parent–child contact over time related to lower recidivism rates for mothers at 6 months post-release. More contact also related to more internalizing symptoms in children, although because of the way the data were collected, it was not possible to disaggregate frequency of face-to-face visits from telephone calls.

Moreover, the addition of assessing cortisol levels via hair samples in the McClure et al. (2015) study allowed for unique insights into relations among incarcerated mothers' contact with children, maternal stress, and maternal and child adjustment, with implications for improved practices and policies. More high quality studies are needed that bring together multiple methodologies, including biological measures, on the phenomena of stress and coping for incarcerated parents and their children and families during and following prison. Such basic research is needed to inform the development of effective interventions that assist families as they raise their children in the face of incarceration, that help incarcerated parents exit criminal lifestyles and avoid future incarceration, and that ultimately keep future generations out of prison or jail and living constructive and fulfilling lives in the community.

5.3 Recommendations

In the following section, I suggest several recommendations that may allow improvements in the experience of parent–child contact during parental incarceration or even improvements in child and parent well-being in the context of parental incarceration. These include suggestions related to parenting interventions, policies and procedures focusing on parent–child contact in corrections facilities, systematic collection of data by corrections systems and more rigorous research in general, and consideration of alternatives to incarceration. It is important to note that when making recommendations about children's contact with incarcerated parents, it is critical to consider the type of corrections facility, type of contact available, children's ages, and the quality and availability of preparation and supports for children, incarcerated individuals, and caregivers around contact issues.

Parenting interventions. Several parenting interventions are available that have shown positive effects on parent–child contact and well as recidivism and other indices of well-being (e.g., Eddy, Martinez, & Burraston, 2013; Shortt, Eddy, Sheeber, & Davis, 2014). Some interventions may be adopted by entire state corrections systems, such as parenting classes offered to inmates or information provided about visits (e.g., Eddy et al., 2013), whereas other interventions are tailored to be implemented more locally depending on resources available and perceived needs. In the former case, the intervention may be standard across state prisons, and inmates and families may know what to expect even when an inmate moves to a different facility. However, in such cases it may be more challenging to provide interventions that are uniquely focused on the culture of or resources available in local communities, where families live. Because jails are locally-operated and located, they may be more accessible for community intervention efforts than prisons, although administrators' openness and ability to change may vary widely and depend on multiple factors across settings.

The McClure et al. (2015) findings regarding benefits of mother-child contact at baseline in prison and mother-child contact after prison are congruent with past findings (Poehlmann et al., 2010), and they support the idea that corrections facilities would do well to identify ways to facilitate positive parent–child contact. There is an accruing literature on how this might be done (Eddy et al., 2013; Loper & Novero, 2010; Shortt et al., 2014), but the field is still in its infancy. To date, what appears to be most promising for incarcerated parents is helping them develop specific cognitive and behavioral skills relevant to emotional regulation and positive parent–child interactions, both inside and outside of the corrections setting. In addition, the findings presented by McClure et al. (2015) suggest the potential added value of more generalized stress management programs with incarcerated parents because of the possible implications for inmate health and functioning as well as for more successful post-release adjustment. This may be particularly true for parents with longer sentences, although these processes need to be studied further in incarcerated fathers.

Such recommendations are consistent with the growing body of literature on programs for incarcerated adults. As Travis and Wahl (2004) have identified, certain parenting interventions, such as behavioral and cognitive skills training, can be effective in reducing recidivism. These interventions are most effective when programs are matched to prisoner risks and needs, well-managed, and supported through post-release supervision. Despite modest reductions in rates of recidivism among participants, Travis and Wahl pointed out that these small reductions can have significant aggregate impacts on criminal behavior in communities with high concentrations of returning prisoners. As noted above, children clearly benefit when formerly incarcerated parents avoid returning to prison or jail and remain positively engaged in children's lives.

Child-friendly visitation. Child-friendly visitation can be defined as providing positive, safe, friendly environments for visits, fostering open communication among caregivers, children, incarcerated parents, and supportive professionals, adequately preparing children for visits, facilitating parent–child contact between visits, and supporting incarcerated parents during the process (Dallaire, Poehlmann, & Loper, 2011). Some parenting interventions in corrections settings offer child-friendly visitation experiences as a component of the intervention (e.g., Parenting Inside Out) whereas some prisons offer child-friendly visits as part of their rehabilitation or parenting programs. For example, the Alleghany County Jail has a family activity center in the jail lobby designed to reduce child stress and provide information to caregivers and includes a craft area for children, videos, books, and miniature mock visiting booths to help prepare children for non-contact visits with jailed parents (Pittsburgh Child Guidance Foundation, 2007). The jail also has a family support center and inmates with children can be selected into a special pod to work with professionals on parenting issues. Given the numbers of children who visit corrections facilities on a daily basis in the United States, it will be important to increase the number of child-friendly visit opportunities available over time in both prisons and jails.

Preparation for visits and providing ample support for children, inmates, and family members during and after visits may have an effect on child or adult behaviors within the context of the corrections institution as well as on child and family well-being. Staff could be trained to learn about children's experiences at jails or prisons and interact with visiting children in a developmentally appropriate manner. It would be helpful if child-friendly materials were available, even something as simple as having a corrections officer give a sticker to a child who has just passed through a metal detector. Corrections staff can be trained more thoroughly in ways of interacting positively with families. Information about visitation could be written or visually depicted in a simple, child-friendly manner and posted at the entry to the jail (e.g., drawings showing the visiting area and the how the hand-held listening device works) as well as on the jail's or prison's website. Five-minute warnings could be given to remind families when the end of the visit is near so children would not be as surprised or distressed by the end of the visit (e.g., a video monitor turning off or the end of a Plexiglas or face-to-face visit). For non-contact visits, barriers between video or Plexiglas booths could be erected so that children are not exposed to other people's visits when talking with their incarcerated parents.

Additional interventions could focus on better preparing caregivers, children, and incarcerated parents for the visit experience, suggesting additional ways for families to stay in touch with an incarcerated parent, and attempting to reduce social stigma associated with parental incarceration, which has recently been conceptualized as a key mechanism for lasting negative effects of parental incarceration on children (Murray, Bijleveld, Farrington, & Loeber, 2014). For example, Sesame Street recently developed materials for young children and their families including an animated depiction of a child's visit to a corrections facility, a story book, videos, and a caregiver guide (*Little Children, Big Challenges: Incarceration,* Sesame Workshop, 2013 http://www.sesamestreet.org/parents/topicsandactivities/toolkits/incarceration). A new Muppet character named Alex was designed for the project. On the video that is part of this project, Alex, who has an incarcerated father, discusses his feelings and experiences in relation to his father's incarceration from a child's point of view. In the video sequences, Alex receives support from an adult and other Muppet characters. The caregiver guide offers suggestions on how families can stay connected with children's incarcerated parents in positive ways, such as writing letters or cards or talking on the phone between visits. The guide also covers topics such as how to talk to very young children about parental incarceration and how to handle some of the common emotional reactions that children may have when their parents go to jail or prison. Sesame Workshop is in the process of evaluating these materials for their efficacy with families affected by parental incarceration, a critical step in the intervention process. Because hard copies of these materials are free and digital copies are widely available on the website (and as a free app for smart phones and tablets), corrections facilities could use them widely to promote healthy child development in the context of parental incarceration.

Policies and procedures in corrections facilities. In the Dallaire et al. (2015) study, more frequent letter-writing and telephone contact were associated with fewer self- and other-reported internalizing behavior problems in school age children.

Internalizing problems such as anxiety, withdrawal, or depression were reported more frequently when children had more barrier visits with their jailed mothers. This finding is consistent with Poehlmann et al.'s (2010) review and suggest that in certain contexts, non-contact visits can be stressful for children. As Poehlmann et al. (2010) have argued, visits may activate a child's attachment system and trigger anxiety that cannot be easily assuaged because the parent–child separation continues following the visit. Poehlmann-Tynan et al.'s findings presented in this monograph show the powerful role that caregivers play during children's non-contact visits with incarcerated parents. More can be done to maximize the positive effects of the caregiver-child relationship within the corrections setting. Moreover, policies and procedures that can help reduce children's anxiety, such as preparing them for visits, maintaining contact between visits, and providing ample support from caregivers and other loved ones before, during and after visits are important for facilitating children's well-being.

It is also interesting to note that children's externalizing (or acting out) problems did not relate to children's contact with incarcerated mothers in the Dallaire et al. (2015) study, neither to letter-writing, telephone contact, nor in-person visits. Although some caregivers have reported concerns about children's acting out behaviors prior to or following visits to corrections facilities, Dallaire et al. (2015) did not replicate this finding. Poehlmann-Tynan et al. (2015) noted increased observer-rated behavioral dysregulation in the jail setting during non-contact visits with incarcerated parents (compared to the home setting), although they did not analyze caregiver-reported behavior problems in this report.

In the Poehlmann-Tynan et al. (2015) study, only one child (of 20 observed) showed overt signs of fear during security procedures at the jail, although many children exhibited periods of serious or somber observation of what was happening around them at the jail. Although physiological measures would be needed to examine children's biological stress response while in the jail setting, adults can still be sensitive to children's needs for reassurance and support during unfamiliar or anxiety-producing experiences. Caregivers can be encouraged to hold children's hands and talk with their children about what the child is seeing and hearing in the corrections settings. Corrections systems can give more information on their websites about policies and procedures relating to security procedures used with children without compromising the safety of the facility, so that caregivers know what to expect when they arrive with child visitors in tow. Corrections staff can be trained to be more supportive of children and families.

Systematic collection of data by corrections systems and rigorous intervention research. In addition to supporting children, caregivers, and incarcerated parents, our research suggests a need for systematic tracking of the number of children affected by parental incarceration and change over time, which could be completed in jail and prison settings as part of the inmate intake or risk assessment process. Inmates can be asked to indicate if they have children and if so, the age of each child. Although some inmates may be reluctant to provide such information because they may fear repercussions from child protective services or intrusion in their private lives by "the system", or they may be in an intoxicated or high state at the time of arrest and intake, many inmates indicate that they are willing to provide such information. Many incarcerated parents are eager to receive parenting support as part of their incarceration and many of them enjoy talking about and finding ways to connect with their children. Such tracking would allow society to more accurately gauge the impact of incarceration on families in communities in each county and state and help determine identification of affected families' needs and allocation of resources.

Rigorous, focused, practical research is also needed on children of incarcerated parents and their families. A key question is how to accomplish such research when funding is tight and such a research agenda does not appear to fit neatly into any one federal agency's funding portfolio. In recognition of this fact, the federal government has pulled together an interagency working subgroup on children with incarcerated parents, which includes diverse departments ranging from the Federal Bureau of Prisons and the Department of Housing and Urban Development to the Department of Health and Human Services (Substance Abuse and Mental Health Services) and disseminates information on the topic http://www.findyouthinfo.gov/youth-topics/children-of-incarcerated-parents. However, even when there is a match between a research agenda and funding portfolio, much of the funding from agencies that could take children of incarcerated parents under their wing goes to programs rather than research. Often funded programs require only a minimal evaluation component. One solution is to form partnerships with state corrections systems to start collecting high quality data on variables that they need to learn about anyway. This could start with inmate risk status, mental health, and contact between inmates and family members, including children, and then expand to conducting low cost randomized controlled trials. It would be even more promising if several states could agree to collect similar data, and test family contact interventions on a systematic basis. Jails could collaborate and follow this model as well.

Consideration of alternatives to incarceration. As I close this chapter, I cannot help but note that the risks associated with mass incarceration that have implications for children and families are well-documented (e.g., Murray et al., 2014). Through short-sighted over-reliance on crime policies used to address challenging social problems, the United States has created a significant and growing public health crisis for its children and has increased racial disparities in health and well-being of children (Wakefield & Wildeman, 2014). Many children who experience the incarceration of a parent are vulnerable and need substantial help now and in the future. These children are at risk for a host of negative outcomes, including the development of antisocial behavior (Murray et al., 2012) as well as long-term health and mental health problems (e.g., Ford et al., 2011). Consideration of alternatives to incarceration may help ease the social and economic burden of corrections on families and society and free up resources that could be used for implementation of preventive interventions to facilitate resilience processes in the next generation.

Acknowledgements When writing this chapter, Dr. Poehlmann-Tynan was supported in part by grants from the National Institutes of Health (R21HD068581, PI: Poehlmann and P30HD03352, PI: Mailick) and the University of Wisconsin. The content is solely the responsibility of the authors and does not necessarily represent the official views of the NIH. Special thanks to J. Mark Eddy, Ph.D., for his input on this chapter.

References

Arditti, J. A., Lambert-Shute, J., & Joest, K. (2003). Saturday morning at the jail: Implications of incarceration for families and children. *Family Relations, 52*(3), 195–204. doi:10.1111/j.1741-3729.2003.00195.x.

Arditti, J. A., & Savla, J. (2013). Parental incarceration and child trauma symptoms in single caregiver homes. *Journal of Child and Family Studies,* 1–11. doi:10.1007/s10826-013-9867-2

Dallaire, D., Poehlmann, J., & Loper, A. (2011). *Issues and recommendations related to children's visitation and contact with incarcerated parents.* United Nations Committee on the Rights of the Child, Day of General Discussion, Children of Incarcerated Parents. http://www2.ohchr.org/english/bodies/crc/discussion2011_submissions.htm

Dallaire, D. H., Zeman, J., & Thrash, T. (2015). Differential effects of type of children's contact with their jailed mothers and children's behavior problems. In J. Poehlmann-Tynan (Ed.), *Children's contact with incarcerated parents: Implications for policy and intervention* (Advances in child and family policy and practice). New York: Springer.

Eddy, J. M., Martinez, C. R., & Burraston, B. (2013). A randomized controlled trial of a parent management training program for incarcerated parents: Proximal impacts. *Monographs of the Society for Research in Child Development, 78*(3), 75–93.

Eddy, J. M., & Poehlmann, J. (Eds.). (2010). *Children of incarcerated parents: A handbook for researchers and practitioners.* Washington, DC: The Urban Institute Press.

Ford, E. S., Anda, R. F., Edwards, V. J., Perry, G. S., Zhao, G., Li, C., et al. (2011). Adverse childhood experiences and smoking status in five states. *Preventive Medicine, 53*(3), 188–193.

Loper, A. B., & Novero, C. (2010). Parenting programs for prisoners. In J. M. Eddy & J. Poehlmann (Eds.), *Children of incarcerated parents: A handbook for researchers and practitioners* (pp. 189–215). Washington, DC: The Urban Institute Press.

McClure, H. H., Shortt, J. W., Eddy, J. M., Holmes, A., Van Uum, S., Russell, E., et al. (2015). Associations among mother-child contact, parenting stress, hair cortisol, and mother and child adjustment related to incarceration. In J. Poehlmann-Tynan (Ed.), *Children's contact with incarcerated parents: Implications for policy and intervention* (Advances in child and family policy and practice). New York: Springer.

Murray, J., Bijleveld, C. C. J. H., Farrington, D. P., & Loeber, R. (2014). *Effects of parental incarceration on children: Cross-national comparative studies.* Washington, DC: American Psychological Association.

Murray, J., Farrington, D. P., & Sekol, I. (2012). Children's antisocial behavior, mental health, drug use, and educational performance after parental incarceration: A systematic review and meta-analysis. *Psychological Bulletin, 138*(2), 175. doi:10.1037/a0026407.

Pittsburgh Child Guidance Foundation. (2007). *Ceremony celebrates opening of "Family Activity Center" at Allegheny County Jail* Retrieved May 10, 2014, from http://foundationcenter.org/grantmaker/childguidance/news-releases-4-21-07.html.

Poehlmann, J., Dallaire, D. H., Loper, A. B., & Shear, L. D. (2010). Children's contact with their incarcerated parents: Research findings and recommendations. *American Psychologist, 65*(6), 575–598. doi:10.1037/a0020279.

Poehlmann, J., & Eddy, J. M. (Eds.) (2013). Relationship processes and resilience in children with incarcerated parents. *Monographs of the Society for Research in Child Development 78* (3, Serial No. 308).

Poehlmann-Tynan, J., Runion, H., Burnson, C., Maleck, S., Weymouth, L., Pettit, K., et al. (2015). Young children's behavioral and emotional reactions to plexiglas and video visits with jailed parents. In J. Poehlmann-Tynan (Ed.), *Children's contact with incarcerated parents: Implications for policy and intervention* (Advances in child and family policy and practice). New York: Springer.

Sesame Workshop and Advisors, Adalist-Estrin, A., Burton, C. F., Gaynes, E., Harris, K. E., & Poehlmann, J. (2013). *Little children, big challenges: Incarceration.* New York: Sesame Workshop.

Shlafer, R. J., Loper, A. B., & Schillmoeller, L. (2015). Introduction and literature review: Is parent-child contact during parental incarceration beneficial? In J. Poehlmann-Tynan (Ed.), *Children's contact with incarcerated parents: Implications for policy and intervention* (Advances in child and family policy and practice). New York: Springer.

Shortt, J. W., Eddy, J. M., Sheeber, L., & Davis, B. (2014). Project home: A pilot evaluation of an emotion-focused intervention for mothers reuniting with children after prison. *Psychological Services, 11*(1), 1. doi:10.1037/a0034323.

The Pew Charitable Trusts. (2010). *Collateral costs: Incarceration's effect on economic mobility*. Washington, DC: Author.

Travis, J., & Wahl, M. (Eds.). (2004). *Prisoners once removed: The impact of incarceration and reentry on children, families, and communities*. Washington, DC: The Urban Institute Press.

Wakefield, S., & Wildeman, C. (2014). *Children of the prison boom: Mass incarceration and the future of American inequality*. Oxford, England: Oxford University Press.

Wildeman, C., & Western, B. (2010). Incarceration in fragile families. *The Future of Children, 20*(2), 157–177.

Chapter 6
Policy Commentary: The Research Evidence Policymakers Need to Build Better Public Policy for Children of Incarcerated Parents

Karen Bogenschneider

This monograph should be commended for taking on the iron law of incarceration—nearly all prisoners come back to their families, neighborhoods, and communities (Travis, 2005). The United States is one of the only countries in the world without a mention of the word *family* in its constitution, so it should come as no surprise that the typical default is to look at policy issues through the lens of the individual with little acknowledgment of the families to which most individuals belong (Bogenschneider, 2014). Political discourse on incarceration is no exception. Attention has focused primarily on the prisoner as an individual without considering the ripple effects that incarceration has on family earnings, family relationships, parenting practices, and child well-being. This collection of papers zeroes in on what may be incarceration's longest-lasting legacy—its impact on the next generation (Kruttschnitt, 2011).

Incarceration rates in the United States have increased sevenfold between the early 1970s and 2010 with an estimated 3 % of the adult population under correctional supervision (Wakefield & Wildeman, 2011). Between 2007 and 2012, prison populations were still increasing in some states, but dropping in others (Arditti, 2014; The Pew Charitable Trusts, 2014). In 2008, inmates confined in county and city jails peaked with a significant decline by 2013 (Golinelli & Minton, 2014). The pendulum of incarceration may have reached its apex, according to Steinberg (2008), as politicians and the public have come to regret the high costs and harshness of penal policy and the ineffectiveness of punitive reforms. Yet the pendulum is likely to move slowly and the effects will not abate any time soon (Wakefield & Wildeman, 2011). Even if incarceration rates returned to 1970 levels, its aftermath will linger on in the

K. Bogenschneider, Ph.D. (✉)
University of Wisconsin-Madison, 4109 Nancy Nicholas Hall,
1300 Linden Drive, Madison, WI, USA
e-mail: kpbogens@wisc.edu

lives of the 2.7 million children outside the prison and jail walls, who are progeny of parents locked inside those walls (Harris & Kearney, 2014). This monograph sheds a bright light on these children—some of society's most vulnerable members—who too often are invisible to those who study and enact incarceration policies.

These comments are targeted to researchers to help clarify what kind of research is most relevant and useful to policymakers, in general, and what evidence is needed to move parental incarceration policy forward, in particular. Too often, policy considerations come up at the back end of a study when researchers are writing their implications. I will suggest here that research could be more policy relevant if policy implications were discussed at the front end of a study when research questions are being formulated, samples selected, measures identified, and analysis designed (Tseng, 2012). I draw on my experience as a knowledge broker connecting policymakers with research knowledge and researchers with policy knowledge on a number of the most important issues of our time. Over the last two decades, my team and I have conducted 33 Wisconsin Family Impact Seminars—a series of presentations, discussion sessions, and briefing reports that communicate high-quality, objective research to state policymakers on topics they identify (see Bogenschneider, 2014). For 15 years, I directed the Family Impact Institute—a network of 26 sites that have convened over 190 Family Impact Seminars for state policymakers across the country, 16 that focused on juvenile or adult crime and 4 that focused specifically on incarceration's impact on children. Not only do I "do" family policy but I "study" it. I have conducted dozens of interviews of state policymakers on what kinds of information they find most useful in their discourse and decisionmaking (Bogenschneider & Corbett, 2010).

Drawing on theory and practice, I drill down on how researchers can become more policy-minded. For policy-informed evidence, I contend that researchers need to understand the policymakers who will be using the information and the environment in which they operate. For evidence-informed policy, I propose that what policymakers need to build better public policy for children of incarcerated parents is evidence that is research-based and family-focused.

6.1 The Political Context in Which Research Is Used

The Family Impact Seminars are built on community dissonance theory, which posits that the underutilization of research in policymaking is due, in large part, to a lack of communication and trust between knowledge producers and knowledge consumers. Researchers and policymakers come from a number of disparate communities that engage in distinct core technologies and operate in diverse professional and institutional cultures with different goals, information needs, languages, and reward systems. Researchers serious about having the findings of their studies used in policy decisions need an understanding of the differences in the institutional cultures in which researchers and policymakers operate (e.g., the pace at which business is conducted, the predominant influences on decisionmaking) and the professional cultures into which they are socialized (e.g., the content that is valued, the vocabulary that is used). Because these cultures shape the way that researchers and policymakers think, act, and perceive the world, they are pervasive, undeniable forces that can facilitate or impede the flow of communication across the research/policy divide. This commentary introduces what the job of policymakers is like and how their work is affected by characteristics of the contemporary lawmaking environment—the partisanship and polarization of policymaking, political support for people in need, and political support for families. Implications are drawn for what each mean for those interested in generating and disseminating policy relevant research on children of incarcerated parents.

6.1.1 The Job of a Policymaker

The core technology of a policymaker is to make laws. Policymaking bodies, like most institutions, have long-standing operational procedures and rules that set powerful constraints on what can and cannot be done (Weiss, 1999). Operating within these institutional parameters, policymakers often use a sifting and winnowing process in order to sort out and make sense of the multitude of ideas that cross their desks. One calculus policymakers apply during this sorting process is what economic benefits will accrue to society for any investments taxpayers make.

What does the nature of a policymaker's job mean for research on parental incarceration? When targeting the information needs of policymakers, it is important to emphasize the outcomes that matter most to them. For example, researchers tend to be more interested in the private value of policies and programs for the individuals and families who participate in them. In contrast, policymakers are more interested in the public value that individuals and families perform for the larger economic and social goals of society. For example, policymakers may be less interested in whether or not ex-offenders reunite with their family, and more interested in how reuniting with their family influences the odds of finding a job or staying off drugs (Kruttschnitt, 2011; Travis, McBride, & Solomon, 2005). Also, if ex-offenders are to reunite with their families and children or successfully reintegrate into society, policymakers will want to know how the costs of rehabilitation and welfare compare to incarceration and foster care (Kruttschnitt, 2011).

Including in research studies outcomes of interest to policymakers is vital. Equally important is understanding how the contemporary lawmaking environment shapes the way research evidence is used.

6.1.2 The Partisanship and Polarization of Policymaking

Amidst questions of how united the United States really is, recent data indicate how far the nation has come apart (Haidt & Hetherington, 2012). Drawing on studies that track Congress over time, partisan polarization was at an all-time low in the 1940s and 1950s; the distance between the parties began to grow in the 1960s and 1970s to the unprecedented divide that exists today. Based on the most current data from 2009, social scientists conclude "it is mathematically impossible for Congress to get much more polarized" (Haidt & Hetherington, 2012, p. 2).

What does this partisan polarization mean for research on parental incarceration? Imagine how the nature of a work environment would change in the face of an opposition whose full-time job it is "to make you look bad" (Levin, 2003, p. 15). Opponents take it upon themselves to closely monitor their colleagues and to meticulously point out any mistakes or misjudgments that can be used against them for political gain in the next election campaign (Levin, 2005). In particular, policymakers' voting records on penal policy may be scrupulously screened for any indication that an opponent is "soft on crime" (Scott & Steinberg, 2008). Given this high level of scrutiny, policymakers will want to know, not only what the research says, but also how much confidence they can have in it. Are these well-accepted, frequently-reported findings or promising new results that need replication? Basically, will the research hold up to the attacks that are sure to come from the other side? For policymakers, it is critical to have information that they can count on to be correct and complete before they present their ideas to colleagues, constituents, and the media. Having the facts right means they are more apt to be re-elected by their constituents and respected by their colleagues in a system that operates on the basis of trust (Bogenschneider & Corbett, 2010).

In the academic culture, the rewards are greater for publishing innovative findings than for replicating findings previously published by others. In the policy culture, innovative findings are of interest, particularly to the most research-minded policymakers (Bogenschneider, Little, & Johnson, 2013) but, in general, policymakers are more apt to value rigorous findings that have been well replicated. For the purposes of this paper, policymakers will need clear and convincing evidence that children benefit or, at a minimum, are not harmed by contacts with incarcerated parents.

As important as understanding how lawmaking bodies operate is recognizing that laws are debated and decided in the midst of a milieu of beliefs and values. Those of particular importance to policy decisions for children of incarcerated parents are political support for people in need and for families.

6.1.3 *Political Support for People in Need*

In recent polls, Americans' support for government programs to help the poor was close to a 25-year low that occurred in 1994. In 2012, only 43 % of Americans believed that government should help more needy people if it meant going deeper into debt, down from 53 % in 1987 and 54 % in 2007. Views on government support for the poor diverge sharply according to political party. Democrats have continued to support government assistance for the poor and needy over the last 25 years, but

Republican support has declined significantly since 2007. In 2012, a minority of Republicans (40 %) agreed that government should take care of people who can't take care of themselves (Pew Research Center, 2012).

What does declining support for people in need mean for research on parental incarceration? These findings imply that it may be difficult to generate bipartisan interest for policies that support those in need, particularly for a group as stigmatized as those ever locked behind bars. However, data that raise the specter of incarceration's impact on children may pique the interest of policymakers, irrespective of their political persuasion. Children are perceived as being placed at-risk because they were thrust into a situation they did not cause and are not responsible for. Beyond the impacts on children, researchers also can factor into their studies the political support that exists for families. Families have proven to be politically popular across the ideological spectrum.

6.1.4 Political Support for Families

Families are considered the cornerstone of a sound economy and a strong society among policymakers, professionals, and the public alike. Policymakers often invoke the language and symbol of *family* because it appeals to common values with the potential to rise above politics (Strach, 2007). For example, a review of the Congressional Record revealed that across a decade, except for 2 weeks, family-oriented words appeared every single week Congress was in session. Importantly, this concern for families did not vary by gender or political party, so the family "brand" has not been captured by the right or left (Strach, 2007). What's more, professionals who educate, administer, or deliver services to families have issued over 50 reports in the last quarter century, calling for family-focused policies, programs, and practices in fields ranging from child care to welfare, from elder care to children of incarcerated parents (see Bogenschneider, 2014; Dunst, Trivette, & Hamby, 2007; Spoth, Kavanagh, & Dishion, 2002). In addition, support for families is widespread among the public, whose views matter to policymakers because it is their constituents who elect and re-elect them to office. The public's near-universal endorsement of families as *very important* to them (94 %; Pew Research Center, 2010) is more than just hollow words. In the 2008 election, the presidential candidates' position on family values were *extremely* or *very important* to how the vast majority of Americans voted—86 % of Republicans, 72 % of Democrats, and 71 % of Independents (Carroll, 2007).

What does political support for families mean for research on parental incarceration? As previously proposed, interest may be piqued in incarceration policy by documenting the problem with data regarding impacts on children, who are seen as deserving recipients of a policy response. However, when it comes to addressing the problem, policymakers will want to know if using family approaches is more effective and cost-efficient than individual approaches as has been widely demonstrated in early childhood education and care, health care, long term care, juvenile crime, substance use, and welfare reform (see Bogenschneider, 2014). For example, studies of foster care placements have compared the effectiveness of a family-focused versus a group-based treatment for delinquent youth. Compared to traditional group care, trained and supported foster parents who recreated the powerful socialization forces of functional family life were much more effective in reducing delinquent acts and serious crimes among even chronic juvenile offenders. In independent analyses, the benefits of the program substantially outweighed the costs (Chamberlain & Reid, 1991).

Building on this background on the context in which policy decisions are made, this commentary turns to what I argue policymakers need to design better incarceration policy—evidence that is research-based and family-focused. Each is discussed in turn below.

6.2 What Research Evidence Policymakers Need for Decisions on Incarceration Policy

As aptly put by Massoglia and Warner, "Effective policy recommendations must flow from scientifically informed and methodologically rigorous research" (2011, p. 856). Incarceration research, which is burdened by the added constraints of studying vulnerable populations in closed environments, suffers from some of the usual shortcomings—biased samples (Arditti, 2012; Wakefield & Wildeman, 2011), non-random assignment of individuals to confinement (Kruttschnitt, 2011), lack of intergenerational data (Wakefield & Wildeman, 2011), self-report measures (McClure et al., in this volume), and so forth. In addition, studies of incarcerated parents suffer from other shortcomings such as the failure to disentangle differences based on the type of contact (e.g., written, phone, video, plexiglass), the source of contacts (e.g., spouses, children, unmarried partners, friends; Holt & Miller, 1972), the confinement sentence and setting (e.g., jail, prison; Poehlmann, Dallaire, Booker Loper, & Shear, 2010); and the intense emotions that can arise when studying families experiencing challenging circumstances (Arditti, Joest, Lambert-Shute, & Walker, 2010). Given these limitations, the literature is plagued with inconsistent findings with research needed on several fronts to provide a "more precise estimate of all the moving parts" (Massoglia & Warner, 2011, p. 823).

Those who study parental incarceration know what rigorous research is and are familiar with the field, so the focus of this section is not to review the literature or the findings reported in this monograph. Instead, this section will identify three research directions that would be useful to policymakers when making decisions on incarceration policy: how children's well-being is influenced by contact with incarcerated parents, which conditions moderate the impact, what mediating pathways influence children for better or worse, and what the cost/benefits might be of intervening in ways that will benefit children.

6.2.1 How Children's Well-Being Is Influenced by Contact with Incarcerated Parents

One of the first questions policymakers are likely to ask is this: Why should children of incarcerated parents be a top policy priority on their legislative agenda amongst the hundreds of issues they are lobbied to take up, often by loud and powerful voices? To exemplify the volume of issues that cross policymakers' desks, in a typical biennium in Wisconsin, there are 1,200 bill requests in the Assembly and 600 in the Senate. With a legislative agenda so crowded, policymakers may be inclined to take notice when confronted with the cost of the U.S. penal system—growing from $7 billion in 1980 to $70 billion in 2007 (Arditti, 2012) and its reach—releasing as many men each year as graduate from college (exactly the type of "social math" that policymakers find useful; Massoglia & Warner, 2011). Before this issue gets any traction though, policymakers will want clear and convincing evidence of whether children are harmed by contact with incarcerated parents, and if so, how serious the harm is. Intuitively, some policymakers are likely to be skeptical, questioning whether some children might actually benefit when an abusive or violent parent is removed from the home.

Wakefield and Wildeman (2011) do not dispute that some children will benefit from the incarceration of their parent, yet provide more precise estimates of child impacts, writ large, using two representative longitudinal data sets with high-quality measurement and several waves of data collection. Multiple modeling strategies allow them to tease apart whether any negative effects on children stem from other sources of childhood disadvantage, in general, or from parent incarceration, in particular. Across all models and data sources, fathers' incarceration appears to increase both externalizing problems (e.g., aggression, delinquency) and internalizing problems (e.g., anxiety, depression) by about one third to one half of a standard deviation. After preexisting disadvantages are accounted for, this translates into approximately a 4–6 % increase in mental health and behavioral problems. A more substantial effect was noted in one data set where levels of physical aggression increased between 19 and 33 %. With this one exception, most of these reported effects are not large, which makes it even more difficult to build the case for lawmakers' attention and action.

A related question is whether these effects are magnified or mitigated when children have contact with parents while they are in prison. One extensive literature review of 36 studies conducted after 1998 concluded that the impact of visitation on parents (with few exceptions) was beneficial. However, the impact on children was mixed with 58 % of studies showing benefits for children and 42 % that did not (Poehlmann et al., 2010). Emerging evidence suggests that an important consideration may be the quality of the contact. In one study, the trauma that children experienced in their visit with incarcerated parents was completely mediated by how problematic and distressing the contact was (Arditti & Savla, 2013). Paralleling this study, the findings reported in this monograph appear to be conditional. It is difficult to draw definitive conclusions across studies that vary in how old the child is, whether the parents are confined in a jail or prison, what type of contact occurred, and so forth.

In sum, the mixed findings suggest that the question may be more complicated than whether or not contact with incarcerated parents affects children's well-being. If policymakers are going to take action, researchers will need to provide more conclusive data on increasingly nuanced questions such as which children are most likely to be affected and under what conditions. The next section examines the value to policymakers of knowing which conditions moderate child impacts.

6.2.2 Which Conditions Moderate the Impact of Children's Contact with Parents

Existing research suggests that child impacts may be conditional depending on the developmental stage of the child (Kruttschnitt, 2011), characteristics of the incarcerated parent (Arditti, 2012; Edin & Nelson, 2013; McKay, Bir, & Lindquist, 2014), the type of contact (Arditti, 2012; Poehlmann et al., 2010), the quality of the contact (Arditti & Savla, 2013), the confinement sentence and setting (Poehlmann et al., 2010), and so forth. For other policy issues, policymakers have found research on moderators to provide useful guidance for policy decisions. As an example, one paper that laid out moderators to consider when developing poverty policy, was almost instantly picked up and used by policymakers. To explain how policymakers could design policies targeted to the disparate needs of diverse segments of the poverty population, Corbett (1993) used an onion analogy. The outer layer of the onion represents those who are plunged into poverty by a discrete event such as divorce or the loss of a job. This subgroup already possesses the skills and motivation to achieve economic self-sufficiency, but may need time-limited and short-term help into the labor market through policies like affordable child care and the Earned Income Tax Credit. The middle layer of the onion represents those with limited options and low earnings capacity. This subgroup has reasonable levels of basic skills and education, but their preparation for the workforce may not match available employment opportunities. To lift this group out of poverty, policies are needed that provide specialized training and vocational education.

Another example of the usefulness of moderators is the differential response approach recently adopted in child protective services. Case workers, sometimes in teams, evaluate reports of maltreatment on a case-by-case basis and typically assign them into one of two or more categories based on imminent danger and risk to a child. The "investigation" category, generally reserved for reports of the most severe types of maltreatment or those that are potentially criminal, require a formal determination or substantiation of child abuse or neglect. The "assessment" category, usually applied in low- and moderate-risk cases, entails a review of the family's strengths and stressors to determine how to address needs and support positive parenting without a formal determination of child abuse or neglect (Abner & Gordon, 2012; Child Welfare Information Child Welfare Information Gateway, 2008).

Researchers have also used statistical techniques like latent class analysis to identify policy-relevant moderators. For example, Courtney and colleagues developed four distinct profiles of young people transitioning from foster care into young adulthood (Courtney, Hook, & Lee, 2010). To respond to each profile's distinct characteristics and needs, specific policies were suggested that could support a successful transition into adulthood.

Similarly, research on moderators could provide useful data to drive decisions on children's contact with incarcerated parents. Profiles could be developed to indicate when contact is and is not advisable depending upon characteristics of the children, the parent, the place and quality of the contact, the support that is provided, and so forth.

Research of this genre can make policymakers confident that the interventions they are funding are being targeted to those who might benefit most. For those that do not benefit, researchers can explore ways to enhance or supplement the intervention or identify alternative approaches that might be more effective. Beyond targeting, it is also helpful for policymakers to know the mediating pathways through which impact occurs.

6.2.3 What Mediating Pathways Influence Children for Better or Worse

Research evidence is also needed on the pathways through which children's contact with parents transmits its influence (Sampson, 2011), which often derive from different theoretical perspectives. Some theories explain if and how family relationships are affected by contact with incarcerated parents, and other theories explain whether policies and programs can repair any harm that results. For example, in one study framed in attachment theory, children who had visited their mother in prison, compared to those who had not, had slightly less positive mental representations of their attachment relationships with their mothers (Poehlmann, 2005). A randomized control trial grounded in social interaction learning theory found that it is possible to improve family relationships by teaching parents behavioral family management skills. Compared to nonparticipants, parents who participated in the program while in prison were less distressed, less depressed, and interacted more positively with their child (Eddy, Martinez, & Burraston, 2013).

Studies framed in risk and resilience theory will resonate with conservative-leaning policymakers, who often express interest in knowing what makes it possible for some individuals to thrive despite adversity. Promising evidence has emerged on processes that promote resilience by protecting children with incarcerated parents from negative consequences; for example, empathy appears to protect children from being rated as aggressive by their classmates (Dallaire & Zeman, 2013) and positive emotion regulation helps children refrain from hostile teasing and bullying (Myers et al., 2013).

Other studies, theorized from a perspective of child trauma, examine whether children's repeated exposure to traumatic circumstances overwhelms their ability to cope (National Child Traumatic Stress Network, 2014). Researchers describe examples of child trauma during visits to incarcerated parents: children banging on the glass barrier separating them from their parent (Arditti, 2012); a child becoming hysterical when he thought his father had no legs because he could only see his body through the glass barrier (Arditti, 2012); following an abrupt ending to a video visit, a child becoming distressed and teary-eyed wondering, "Where did Daddy go?" (see Poehlmann et al., this volume); and so forth. Heart-wrenching stories of trauma can be useful to policymakers for making persuasive political arguments, but what is even more useful is evidence on how pervasive and potent these traumatic events are.

Research on the mediating mechanisms that link incarceration to children's outcomes are valuable to policymakers in a couple ways. First, the old maxim that "nothing is as practical as a good theory" is as true for policymakers as it is for researchers. Theories are useful to policymakers by making explicit their (often implicit) assumptions about why children may be harmed or helped by contact with incarcerated parents. Theories can serve to alter the terms of policy debate by providing policymakers with a conceptual framework and a common language for thinking about problems and designing policy responses (Bogenschneider & Gross, 2004).

Second, because different mediators drive different policy responses, this line of inquiry can provide guidance to policymakers who face "up or down" votes on dramatically divergent policy options (Massoglia & Warner, 2011). For example, would it be most effective for policymakers to intervene at the child level to build resilience or to reduce children's exposure to trauma? Or should policymakers support family approaches and, if so, would it be most effective to focus on the relationship level to improve attachment security or on the behavioral level to improve parenting behaviors and family management skills?

As researchers, we have the luxury of delving deeply into specific issues. Policymakers, however, are put in the unenviable position of having to weigh every issue against all the others clamoring for attention, and prioritize those which warrant an infusion of public resources. Knowing how policymakers set priorities can be informative for conducting policy relevant research.

6.2.4 What the Cost/Benefits Are of Intervening in Ways That Will Benefit Children

Policymakers face constraints that researchers can largely ignore in their work, none more important than budgetary realities. The job of the policymaker involves responding to the demand from constituents (which is unrelenting) for resources (which are always in short supply). Policymakers are elected to allocate resources as fairly and efficiently as possible in ways that improve the economic and social well-being of society. For penal policy, data that would be useful to policymakers are economic estimates of the "full ramifications of incarceration's costs and benefits" (Sampson, 2011, p. 824). Policymakers find themselves forced to balance the benefits of incarceration (such as crimes averted) against the costs (such as the compromised human capital development of the children of incarcerated parents). Granted, quantifying the costs and benefits of incarceration is hard, but just because it is hard does not mean that it is not worth doing. When it can be done, a dollars and cents argument can be powerful.

One recent example of the power of economic data in shaping prison policy comes from the state of Washington. Policymakers were worried about the exorbitant cost of building another prison. They asked the Washington State Institute for Public Policy to conduct a meta-analysis of the cost effectiveness of 571 rigorously evaluated criminal justice programs. A net benefit was calculated for each program by subtracting the program's costs from imputed benefits to taxpayers and crime victims (who were spared monetary costs and reduced quality of life). The researchers found that some programs saved the state thousands of dollars, whereas others cost the state more money than they saved. Using this analysis, the state decided not to build another prison. Instead, they invested in the five most cost-beneficial rehabilitation programs and the single most cost-beneficial prevention program. These six programs yield net benefits that range from a low of $12,822 for each dollar spent to a high of $77,798. These dramatic savings illustrate quite vividly the potential of policies and programs for incarcerated parents to show substantial net benefits given the high costs of victimization and the justice system.

The most cost-effective programs were the ones that focused on juveniles, all which used family, rather than individual, approaches (Aos, Miller, & Drake, 2006). This finding reinforces the importance of examining policy for incarcerated parents through the lens of family impact.

6.3 What Family-Focused Research Policymakers Need for Decisions on Incarceration Policy

Ironically, the issue of *family* was relatively invisible in studies of incarceration until researchers began framing their work in economic theory, using the concepts of *collateral costs* and *externality*. The idea of externality—the costs or benefits to a person who did not choose to incur that cost or benefit—made explicit the connections between prison and parenthood across a number of macro disciplines like criminology, demography, and sociology (Arditti, 2014). Research evidence on the collateral costs of incarceration has documented the "intergenerational transmission of class disadvantage and racial disparities," prompting scholars to begin calling for Family and Children Impact Statements to accompany all penal policies (Comfort, Nurse, McKay, & Kramer, 2011, p. 845; Shedd, 2011).

This idea of viewing policies and programs through the lens of their impact on families is not new, dating back to the 1976 U.S. Senate subcommittee hearings on the state of American families chaired by Senator Walter Mondale (Ooms, 1995). Almost four decades ago, testimony by distinguished scholars such as Urie Bronfenbrenner, Margaret Mead, and Edward Zigler called for family impact statements that, like environmental impact statements, would routinely assess the impact of government policies and programs on family well-being. In response, the Family Impact Seminar (FIS) was formed at George Washington University and was charged with studying family impact statements as an approach for prioritizing families in policy and practice decisions.

After conducting three in-depth national studies and 12 community-level field projects, the Family Impact Seminars argued against establishing a formal family impact statement mechanism, fearing that it might be highly regulatory and intrusive (Ooms & Preister, 1988). Instead, a broader family impact framework was recommended that included a range of tools and educational strategies to help policymakers analyze whether viewing issues through the lens of family impact would result in more effective and efficient policy responses and what the consequences of any program or policy might be for family well-being. This broader vision of promoting the family impact lens in policymaking has been kept alive by the Policy Institute for Family Impact Seminars, recently renamed the Family Impact Institute (Bogenschneider et al., 2012). A new theoretical and empirical rationale is available as well as a handbook with pragmatic processes and procedures for applying the family impact lens at the time policies are enacted, when programs are established, and when practices are implemented (see the family impact section of the website at www.familyimpactseminars.org).

At the heart of the family impact lens is understanding the sweeping changes that have occurred in the lives of fragile families. Many policymakers and professionals who regulate families are not familiar with research on the demographic changes that disadvantaged families are experiencing, particularly partner instability, multipartner fertility, and unwed parenthood. This section begins by describing family life in contemporary fragile families and then illustrates how using the lens of family impact can guide researchers and policymakers in their efforts to build better public policy for children of incarcerated parents.

6.3.1 The Sweeping Changes in the Lives of Contemporary Fragile Families

Researchers often caution that it is important not to view families with an incarcerated member through a deficit perspective that can inadvertently blind one to the strengths they possess (McHale, Salman, Strozier, & Cecil, 2013). Similarly, viewing fragile families through more advantaged, middle-class eyes can inadvertently blind one to how parenthood is being redefined by disadvantaged, unmarried fathers. This section draws on quantitative and qualitative data on fragile families with the caveat that all incarcerated parents are not alike, particularly those serving sentences in prisons and jails. The quantitative data derives from an ongoing longitudinal study of 1,479 couples in which the male partner was incarcerated in a state prison with an average sentence of 6.5 years (personal communication from Tasseli McKay, September 12, 2014). The family structures were complex with the typical man fathering children with three different women, and the women typically co-parenting with two different men. Before incarceration, over two thirds of the fathers had lived with at least one child before being married and the majority (60 %) had children they did not live with (McKay et al., 2014).

A recent qualitative study provides a more in-depth look at the complexity of family life in these fragile families. Edin and Nelson (2013) conducted 2 years of ethnographic fieldwork followed by 5 years of repeated in-depth interviews across a number of low-income Philadelphia neighborhoods (a "must read" for anyone studying or working with fragile families). To collect this data, the researchers and their children lived in a two-room apartment in the Rosendale neighborhood of East Camden. In this neighborhood, as in many like them across the country, steady work and decent wages have become increasingly out-of-reach (Cherlin, 2009) amidst social structures that increasingly disenfranchise disadvantaged men from any positive role in society (Edin & Nelson, 2013).

For these low-income men, rarely is pregnancy deliberately planned or actively avoided. Couples do not "'fall in love,' get engaged, or get married before conceiving a first child together" (Edin & Nelson, 2013, p. 32). The norm is that couples are "together" a couple months before the child is conceived. The news that a man is going to become a father is the time when the real relationship building with the mother begins. The prospect of becoming a father is greeted joyfully with a burst of optimism and enthusiastic plans to stay involved in the child's life. At first, these plans materialize with about 80 % of the fathers in a romantic relationship with the mother when the baby is born, and about half still with her when the baby turns one. But by the time of the child's fifth birthday, there is less than a one in three chance that the biological parents will still be together.

The way it used to be was that men were partners first and fathers second. The way it is now for disadvantaged fathers is that the child is at the center and the mother is on the periphery. For these men, fathering a child, even one they can't financially support, is viewed as a chance to accomplish something of lasting value. It is hard to fathom a "life so devoid of good news that an unplanned pregnancy and the birth of a baby—a child one can't possibly support—is viewed as a blessing" (Edin & Nelson, 2013, p. 188). These men are willing to invest a great deal in their relationships with their children, but are hesitant to invest too much in the relationship with the child's mother. This puts the father at high risk for what has now become the statistical norm—multiple partner fertility. Mothers are most often the custodial parent, so when fathers fail in one romantic relationship, they will try again to be a good father to another child with another mother. Fathering another child may occur because it is "better to be a great dad to one kid, particularly one he hasn't failed yet, rather than a so-so dad to all of his kids" (Edin & Nelson, 2013, p. 187).

Being a good father is defined by these men, less by providing for them financially, and more by being there for them emotionally, a role they can more realistically fulfill. Despite all the impediments they face, about 70 % of disadvantaged fathers manage to stay intensively involved in the lives of one of their children. However, the financial and emotional resources that fathers have to give are not spread out evenly, with more money and time going to their younger than older children.

Fragile families become more complicated when the mother finds a new partner. Sometimes she gives the new man the title of "daddy" of her children to reward him for his contributions, which are voluntary, and to signal to the biological father how meager his economic support is. Thus, some disadvantaged men play a larger role as fathers to their partner's children than to some of their own biological children.

For those studying and designing policy for incarcerated parents, it is important to consider the implications of these changing family norms among fragile families. Only three implications are considered here—what the advertent and inadvertent consequences are for families, who the concept of family should include, and whether family disparities exist.

6.3.2 What Advertent and Inadvertent Consequences Incarceration Policy Has for Families

Incarceration policy has many consequences for families, some that are intended, but many that are not. One telling example was the passage of President Clinton's 1977 Adoption and Safe Families Act. The law had an admirable goal—reducing the number of children living in unsafe homes or foster care. To this end, states were required to terminate the parental rights of children who had been in foster care for 15 of the past 22 months. However, given that the mean sentence for drug offenses was 31 months, this law resulted in more incarcerated parents (mostly mothers) having their parental rights terminated, a consequence that lawmakers may not have intended (Kruttschnitt, 2011; Shedd, 2011). Considering this law through the lens of family impact would likely have made this consequence explicit, so it could have been factored into the debate before the decision was finalized.

Research and policy on prisons or jails, if subjected to a family impact analysis, could identify family impacts such as how far institutions are located from families, how easy or hard it is to locate visitation policies on the website, how much time is allowed for visits, whether children are subjected to screening and frisking, and what the conditions are surrounding the visit (e.g., privacy of contact, availability of books and toys). Law enforcement research and policy, if viewed through the family impact lens, would be more cognizant of the (well-documented) ways in which the arrest of a parent is traumatizing for a child (Shedd, 2011). The prevalence of children witnessing the arrest of their parent ranges from estimates of 20 % to over 84 % (Arditti, 2012). Yet even when the child was present during the arrest, only about four of ten officers (42 %) asked who would be available to care for the child (Kruttschnitt, 2011).

Another set of criminal sanctions, often referred to as invisible punishments (Travis et al., 2005), stem from the impact of a number of state statutes and administrative rules on prisoners after their release. Many of these invisible punishments affect returning prisoners and their families (e.g., whether or not a prisoner can access food pantries or homeless shelters, obtain a driver's license or voter ID, or qualify for benefits such as food stamps or health care). Recently, some states have lifted restrictions that may ease an ex-offender's transition back to their family, neighborhood, and community. As of 2009, 30 states now allow ex-prisoners to receive food stamps or welfare assistance if they meet certain conditions (e.g., passing drug tests, participating in treatment) and 9 states have no conditions at all. Yet 11 states still ban welfare benefits in full (Arditti, 2012). Qualitative and quantitative research on the impact of such bans on children's well-being, and on relatives who are forced to choose between severing ties with an ex-offender or losing needed benefits (Comfort et al., 2011) can be useful data for policy decisions. Beyond these consequences, the family impact lens also can broaden the focus beyond the prisoner to his or her family, a topic explored more fully in the next section.

6.3.3 *Who the Concept of Family Should Include*

When a family impact lens is used, the family is treated as a holistic unit, which suggests acknowledging kin and other close relationships (Comfort et al., 2011). For children with an incarcerated parent, the focus is often on the parent/child dyad even though the caregiver functions as a co-parent, and often has more control over contact with the child than a judge or social worker (Poehlmann et al., 2010). A family impact perspective would suggest moving beyond the dyad to a triad or even a family-wide assessment of the parenting a child is receiving (McHale et al., 2013). Also, despite the fact that aunts and uncles play important parenting roles in some cultures, the value of kin relationships is not reflected in prison policies. In South Carolina, as an example, a niece or nephew can visit only if the inmate has been behind bars for three consecutive years (Acock & Acock, 2014).

The family impact lens would also suggest that researchers interested in children of incarcerated parents consider targeting interventions to the marital or couple relationship. Drawing on studies of parental education, longitudinal randomized control trials have compared the effects of a parent-focused versus couple-focused approach. Compared to the control group, couples in the parent-focused group were more effective in their interactions with their children 1 year later; however, no changes were observed in the quality of the couple relationship. Notably, for the parents in the couple-focused group, both the parent–child and couple relationship improved. The children showed higher academic achievement and lower aggression in first grade, and continued to show better school performance and fewer problem behaviors 10 years later when they transitioned into high school. Also, parents in the couple-focused group experienced a decline in depression, marital conflict, and parenting stress (Cowan & Cowan, 2008).

Researchers and policymakers sometimes fail to recognize the complexity of ways that fragile families are structured and function. For example, incarcerated men may be serving as a father to children they do not have a biological relationships with. In one institution, fathers were permitted to put only one girlfriend on their list of visitors. This "one girlfriend policy" forces fathers to choose which of their children they want to see (Arditti, 2012). Beyond these effects on individual prisoners, the family impact lens can indicate impacts on whole subgroups of people, as illustrated next.

6.3.4 *Whether Family Disparities Exist*

Consistent with a family impact perspective, researchers have well documented the disparate family impacts of the incarcerated population, which is overwhelmingly poor, male, and minority. Wide disparities exist between Whites and African Americans and, in recent studies, Hispanics as well (Arditti, 2012). Using data that provides an historical perspective on racial disparities, African American children born in 1990 had a 25.1 % risk that their father would be imprisoned by their 14th birthday, compared to only 3.6 % for White children (Wakefield & Wildeman, 2011). Using current data, children born to an African American father without a high school diploma face a 50 % odds their father will be behind bars by their 14th birthday (Harris & Kearney, 2014). Researchers also have documented the real-world consequences of these racial disparities for children of incarcerated parents. Absent incarceration, the Black-White disparities in children's internalized behavior problems would have been 25–45 % smaller and the Black-White disparities in externalized behavior problems would have been 14–26 % smaller (Wakefield & Wildeman, 2011).

Why policymakers have not addressed these deepening race and class disparities can be attributed to several factors, one that is of special significance to researchers. In today's polarized policy context, policymakers may be unwilling to introduce corrective legislation that puts their name (and credibility) on the line unless they have confidence that it will work. What policymakers need is rigorous and reliable data on the ways in which disparities are created, why they are perpetuated, and how they can be attenuated. Researchers could contribute to addressing disparities by examining differential treatment at every point in the criminal justice process—pretrial, arrest, prosecution, and adjudication (Arditti, 2012).

6.4 Discussion

Researchers are often criticized by policymakers and by knowledge brokers for their caution in concluding that more research is needed. As a knowledge broker, I find myself agreeing with the cautious conclusion of Kruttschnitt (2011) that more research is needed to build evidence-informed policy for children of incarcerated parents: "We should intervene in this policy arena only when we have considered creatively and carefully what will be required to make a difference in the lives of children of incarcerated parents" (p. 835). In the academic culture, this monograph highlights many of the important inroads that researchers are making step-by-step, study-by-study. In the policy culture, where policymakers are forced to take an "up" or "down" vote, the verdict still appears to be out on whether to enact and fund policies and programs that encourage children's contact with incarcerated parents. Policymakers shy away from issues with ambiguous research results, so classic experiments may be called for to cut through the fog of conflicting and confusing evidence (see Eddy et al., 2013).

For researchers, this means opportunities abound for producing research-based, family-focused evidence to build better public policy for children of incarcerated parents. Policymakers need a more complete and comprehensive understanding of the consequences of children's contact with incarcerated parents, what the mediators and moderators of that influence are, and what the cost/benefits might be of taking steps to sever the legacy of incarceration for the next generation.

Policymakers need a better grasp of how contemporary families are affected by and adapting to changing cultural, economic, and social conditions so that policy and practice decisions can be better targeted to the complexity of the way fragile families are structured and function. Policymakers need to know more about the conditions of confinement, a line of inquiry that is disappearing (with the exception of studies of super-max prisons; Kruttschnitt, 2011). Despite the importance of this genre of research on child impacts, it may be equally important for researchers to move upstream and study how we can lower the high rates of placing people behind lock and key, reduce the race and class disparities that exist, and rebuild the circumstances and life chances of society's most fragile families that prime them for the prison pipeline.

Research on incarceration, no matter how good, has a better chance of influencing policy decisions when it is designed and communicated in policy-relevant ways that emphasize how actions to protect children and reunite former offenders with their families benefit the larger social and economic goals of society. For example, prison/jail administrators are often resistant to participate in studies or release secondary data (J. Arditti, personal communication, July 29 2014), so researchers may need to better communicate how the data can be useful for cutting costs, improving inmate behavior, and/or reducing recidivism. Also, in today's polarized policymaking environment, it is more important than ever to emphasize the rigor of the research and how much confidence we can have in the findings. Policymakers need to know what the collateral consequences are for children and how these consequences are shaped by moderating and mediating influences.

Given the field's mixed findings on how children's well-being is influenced by contact with incarcerated parents, researchers need to examine moderating influences such as which children are most likely to be helped or harmed by contact with their parents (Kruttschnitt, 2011) and under what conditions these effects occur (Poehlmann et al., 2010). As has proven useful for other social policy issues, researchers need to look beyond individual markers of risk and resilience to create typologies or profiles of a number of characteristics of the child, the parent, the contact, the confinement setting, and so forth that identify the conditions under which children do better or worse. On other policy issues, researchers have met this challenge by identifying profiles of moderating influences using quantitative methods such as latent class analysis (Courtney et al., 2010) and qualitative methods such as syntheses of literature reviews and meta-analysis (Corbett, 1993).

Policy decisions would also benefit from research on what processes mediate the influence that contact with incarcerated parents has on children and the theoretical mechanisms whereby these effects occur. Theories can be extraordinarily useful to policymakers because they can provide a common language for conceptualizing the issue that can steer policymakers toward specific policy responses such as efforts to build resilience at the child level, strengthen parenting practices or attachment relationships at the parent level, modify the types or conditions of the parent/child contact at the institution level, and so forth. However, as Sampson (2011) points out, complexity reigns supreme. There is no sole effect on children in one discrete developmental domain, so there is not likely to be a single, sacrosanct policy response that is the "silver bullet" that policymakers often yearn for. The task that looms ahead for researchers is tackling a complex issue with nuanced thinking, rigorous methods, and sophisticated analyses to identify the multiple and variable pathways through which children's contact with incarcerated parents transmits its influence.

This commentary identifies several ways that viewing children's contact with incarcerated parents through the lens of family impact can indicate multiple, often inadvertent consequences of policies, programs, and practices for children and families. Typically, family impact analysis entails a qualitative process of drawing from existing evidence to estimate likely consequences. However, it could consist of conducting an in-depth empirical analysis or computer simulation to document how widespread the disadvantages are for families, how consequential and long-lasting they are, and how cost effective it would be to develop and implement policies, programs, and practices that are more family friendly.

It seems appropriate to end a policy commentary with a challenge from a politician that appears as relevant today as when it was issued in 1903. The 26th President of the United States, Teddy Roosevelt, challenged us to a level of greatness that rises to the level of our opportunity (Morris, 2001). For researchers, a tremendous opportunity lies ahead to generate research evidence that can make a difference in the lives of some of society's most vulnerable members. The number of children losing a parent to incarceration and being exposed to the penal system is unprecedented. Similarly, the academic community is called to produce research-based, family-focused evidence for policymakers that is unprecedented in its scale and quality.

Acknowledgements Sincere appreciation is expressed to Joyce Arditti, Tom Corbett, and Michael Massoglia for their insightful comments on an earlier draft of this manuscript.

References

Abner, K., & Gordon, R. A. (2012). *Differential response: A family impact analysis* (Family impact analysis series). Madison, WI: Family Impact Institute.

Acock, A. C., & Acock, D. A. (2014). When men are released from prison: What have we done? *Family Focus, 59*(F3), F5.

Aos, S., Miller, M., & Drake, E. (2006). *Evidenced-based public policy options to reduce future prison construction, criminal justice costs, and crime rates*. Olympia, WA: Washington State Institute for Public Policy.

Arditti, J. A. (2012). *Parental incarceration and the family: Psychological and social effects of imprisonment on children, parents, and caregivers*. New York: New York University Press.

Arditti, J. A. (2014). A family perspective on incarceration and criminal justice involvement. *Family Focus, 59*, F1–F2, F4, F6–F7.

Arditti, J. A., Joest, K. S., Lambert-Shute, J., & Walker, L. (2010). The role of emotions in fieldwork: A self-study of family research in a corrections setting. *The Qualitative Report, 15*, 1387–1414.

Arditti, J. A., & Savla, J. (2013). Parental incarceration and child trauma symptoms in single caregiver homes. *Journal of Child and Family Studies*, 1–11. doi:10.1007/s10826-013-9867-2

Bogenschneider, K. (2014). *Family policy matters: How policymaking affects families and what professionals can do* (3rd ed.). New York: Routledge and Taylor & Francis Group.

Bogenschneider, K., & Corbett, T. (2010). *Evidence-based policymaking: Insights from policy-minded researchers and research-minded policymakers*. New York: Taylor & Francis Group.

Bogenschneider, K., & Gross, E. (2004). From ivory tower to state house: How youth theory can inform youth policymaking. *Family Relations, 53*, 21–26. doi:10.1111/j.1741-3729.2004.00005.x.

Bogenschneider, K., Little, O., Ooms, T., Benning, S., Cadigan, K., & Corbett, T. (2012). The family impact lens: A family-focused, evidence-informed approach to policy and practice. *Family Relations, 61*, 514–531. doi:10.1111/j.1741-3729.2012.00704.x.

Bogenschneider, K., Little, O., & Johnson, K. (2013). Policymakers' use of social science research: Looking within and across policy actors. *Journal of Marriage and Family, 75*(2), 263–275. doi:10.1111/jomf.12009.

Carroll, J. (2007, December 26). Public: "Family values" important to presidential vote. *Gallup poll*. Retrieved from http://www.gallup.com/poll/103375/public-family-values-important-presidential-vote.aspx

Chamberlain, P., & Reid, J. B. (1991). Using a specialized foster care community treatment model for children and adolescents leaving the state mental hospital. *Journal of Community Psychology, 19*, 266–276. doi:10.1002/1520-6629(199107)19:3<.0.CO;2-5.

Cherlin, A. J. (2009). *The marriage-go-round: The state of marriage and the family in America today*. New York: Knopf.

Child Welfare Information Gateway. (2008). *Differential response to reports of child abuse and neglect*. Retrieved from https://www.childwelfare.gov/pubs/issue_briefs/differential_response/differential_response.pdf

Comfort, M., Nurse, A. M., McKay, T., & Kramer, K. (2011). Taking children into account. *Criminology & Public Policy, 10*, 839–850. doi:10.1111/j.1745-9133.2011.00750.x.

Corbett, T. (1993). Child poverty and welfare reform: Progress or paralysis? *Focus, 15*(1), 1–46.

Courtney, M. E., Hook, J. L., & Lee, J. S. (2010). *Distinct subgroups of former foster youth during young adulthood: Implications for policy and practice* (Issue Brief). Retrieved from http://www.chapinhall.org/sites/default/files/publications/Midwest_IB4_Latent_Class_2.pdf

Cowan, P., & Cowan, C. P. (2008). Diverging family policies to promote children's well-being in the UK and US: Some relevant data from family research and intervention studies. *Journal of Children's Services, 3*(4), 4–16.

Dallaire, D. H., & Zeman, J. L. (2013). Empathy as a protective factor for children with incarcerated parents. *Monographs of the Society for Research in Child Development, 78*, 7–25. doi:10.1111/mono.12018.

Dunst, C. J., Trivette, C. M., & Hamby, D. W. (2007). Meta-analysis of family-centered help-giving practices research. *Mental Retardation and Developmental Disabilities Research Reviews, 13*, 370–378. doi:10.1002/mrdd.20176.

Eddy, J. M., Martinez, C. R., Jr., & Burraston, B. (2013). A randomized controlled trial of a parent management training program for incarcerated parents: Proximal impacts. *Monographs of the Society for Research in Child Development, 78*, 75–93. doi:10.1111/mono.12022.

Edin, K., & Nelson, T. J. (2013). *Doing the best I can: Fatherhood in the inner city.* Berkeley: University of California Press.

Golinelli, D., & Minton, T. D. (2014). *Jail inmates at midyear 2013—Statistical tables* (revised) [Table]. Retrieved from http://www.bjs.gov/index.cfm?ty=pbdetail&iid=4988

Haidt, J., & Hetherington, M. J. (2012, September 17). Look how far we've come apart. *The New York Times.* Retrieved from http://campaignstops.blogs.nytimes.com/2012/09/17/look-how-far-weve-come-apart/

Harris, B. H., & Kearney, M. S. (2014). *The unequal burden of crime and incarceration on America's poor.* Washington, DC: Brookings Institution.

Holt, N., & Miller, D. (1972). *Explorations in inmate-family relationships* (Research Report No. 46). Retrieved from http://www.fcnetwork.org/reading/holt-miller/holt-millersum.html#SUMMARY

Kruttschnitt, C. (2011). Is the devil in the details? Crafting policy to mitigate the collateral consequences of parental incarceration. *Criminology & Public Policy, 10*, 829–837. doi:10.1111/j.1745-9133.2011.00732.x.

Levin, B. R. (2003, November). *Improving research–policy relationships: Lessons from the case of literacy.* Paper prepared for the OISE/UT International Literacy Conference: Literacy Policies for the Schools We Need, Toronto, Canada.

Levin, B. R. (2005). *Governing education.* Toronto, Canada: University of Toronto Press. (Original work published 1952)

Massoglia, M., & Warner, C. (2011). The consequences of incarceration: Challenges for scientifically informed and policy-relevant research. *Criminology & Public Policy, 10*, 851–863. doi:10.1111/j.1745-9133.2011.00754.x.

McHale, J. P., Salman, S., Strozier, A., & Cecil, D. K. (2013). Triadic interactions in mother–grandmother coparenting systems following maternal release from jail. *Monographs of the Society for Research in Child Development, 78*, 57–74. doi:10.1111/mono.12021.

McKay, T., Bir, A., & Lindquist, C. (2014). Facing incarceration and preparing for reentry: The needs and hopes of young families. *Family Focus, 59*(F7), F9–F10.

Morris, E. (2001). *Theodore rex.* New York: Random House.

Myers, B. J., Mackintosh, V. H., Kuznetsova, M. I., Lotze, G. M., Best, A. M., & Ravindran, N. (2013). Teasing, bullying, and emotion regulation in children of incarcerated mothers. *Monographs of the Society for Research in Child Development, 78*, 26–40. doi:10.1111/mono.12019.

National Child Traumatic Stress Network. (2014). *Understanding child trauma.* Retrieved from http://www.nctsn.org/sites/default/files/assets/pdfs/policy_and_the_nctsn_final.pdf

Ooms, T. (1995, October). *Taking families seriously: Family impact analysis as an essential policy tool.* Paper presented at the Expert Meeting on Family Impact, University of Leuven, Leuven, Belgium.

Ooms, T., & Preister, S. (1988). *A strategy for strengthening families: Using family criteria in policymaking and program evaluation.* Washington, DC: AAMFT Research and Education Foundation.

Pew Research Center. (2010). *The decline of marriage and rise of new families.* Retrieved from http://pewsocialtrends.org/files/2010/11/pew-social-trends-2010-families.pdf

Pew Research Center. (2012). *Partisan polarization surges in Bush, Obama years–Trends in American values: 1987–2012* [Press release]. Retrieved from http://www.people-press.org/2012/06/04/partisan-polarization-surges-in-bush-obama-years/

Poehlmann, J. (2005). Representations of attachment relationships in children of incarcerated mothers. *Child Development, 76*, 679–696. doi:10.1111/j.1467-8624.2005.00871.x.

Poehlmann, J., Dallaire, D., Booker Loper, A., & Shear, L. (2010). Children's contact with their incarcerated parents: Research findings and recommendations. *American Psychologist, 65*, 575–598. doi:10.1037/a0020279.

Sampson, R. J. (2011). The incarceration ledger: Toward a new era in assessing societal consequences. *Criminology & Public Policy, 10*, 819–828. doi:10.1111/j.1745-9133.2011.00756.x.

Scott, E. S., & Steinberg, L. D. (2008). *Rethinking juvenile justice*. Cambridge, MA: Harvard University Press.

Shedd, C. (2011). Countering the carceral continuum: The legacy of mass incarceration. *Criminology & Public Policy, 10*, 865–871. doi:10.1111/j.1745-9133.2011.00748.x.

Spoth, R. L., Kavanagh, K. A., & Dishion, T. (2002). Family-centered preventive intervention science: Toward benefits to larger populations of children, youth, and families. *Prevention Science, 3*, 145–152. doi:10.1023/A:1019924615322.

Steinberg, L. (2008). Introducing the issue. *The Future of Children, 18*(2), 3–14.

Strach, P. (2007). *All in the family: The private roots of American public policy*. Stanford, CA: Stanford University Press.

The Pew Charitable Trusts. (2014). *U.S. imprisonment rate continues to drop amid falling crime rates* [Press release]. Retrieved from http://www.pewtrusts.org/en/about/news-room/press-releases/2014/03/14/us-imprisonment-rate-continues-to-drop-amid-falling-crime-rates.

Travis, J. (2005). *But they all come back: facing the challenges of prisoner reentry*. Washington, DC: The Urban Institute Press.

Travis, J., McBride, E. C., & Solomon, A. L. (2005). *Families left behind: The hidden costs of incarceration and reentry*. Washington, DC: The Urban Institute Press.

Tseng, V. (2012). The uses of research in policy and practice. *SRCD Social Policy Report, 26*(2), 1, 3–16.

Wakefield, S., & Wildeman, C. (2011). Mass imprisonment and racial disparities in childhood behavioral problems. *Criminology & Public Policy, 10*, 791–792. doi:10.1111/j.1745-9133.2011.00741.x.

Weiss, C. H. (1999). Research–policy linkages: How much influence does social science research have? In *UNESCO, World Social Science report 1999* (pp. 194–205). Paris: UNESCO.

Index

C
Children, 1–3, 6, 8–18, 23–37, 39–57, 59–62, 64–68, 70, 72–79, 83–90, 93–110
Contact, 1–18, 23–37, 40, 41, 43, 44, 47, 48, 51–54, 59–79, 83–90, 96, 98–102, 106, 107, 109, 110
Corrections, 2–14, 16, 17, 39–41, 45–47, 51–53, 60, 61, 64, 66, 75, 83–90, 93
Cortisol, 18, 62–64, 66, 68–74, 76–79, 86

I
Incarceration, 1–18, 23–26, 35, 36, 39–44, 53, 54, 59–79, 83–86, 88–90, 93–110
Internalizing behavior, 29, 30, 32–35, 88

J
Jail, 1–6, 10, 12–15, 17, 18, 23–37, 39–54, 83–90, 93, 94, 98, 100, 105, 106, 109

M
Maternal incarceration, 24, 25, 35, 36, 60
Mother–child contact, 18, 35, 59–79, 87
Mothers, 1, 10, 12, 14–18, 23–37, 43, 46, 50, 51, 59–79, 85–87, 89, 101, 105, 106

N
Non-contact visits, 8, 18, 24, 37, 53, 54, 85, 87–89

P
Parent–child contact, 1–18, 53, 61, 83–87, 110
Parent–child relationships, 8, 40, 78
Parenting, 2, 11, 12, 14, 15, 18, 53, 59–79, 86, 87, 90, 93, 100, 102, 105, 107, 108, 110
Policy, 2, 3, 8, 10, 12, 16–18, 41, 51, 53, 76, 78, 83, 86, 88–90, 93–110
Prison, 1–3, 6–12, 14–17, 24, 35, 40–42, 45, 52, 54, 59–70, 72, 74–79, 83–90, 93, 94, 98–101, 103, 105–107, 109

R
Reunification, 54, 67, 77, 78, 85

S
Stress, 15, 18, 25, 51, 52, 54, 59–79, 85–87, 89, 102, 108

V
Video visits, 3, 7, 8, 10, 13, 14, 18, 39–54, 84, 102

Made in the USA
Middletown, DE
19 January 2017